Fertility Issues

Editor: Tracy Biram

Volume 387

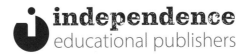
independence
educational publishers

First published by Independence Educational Publishers

The Studio, High Green

Great Shelford

Cambridge CB22 5EG

England

© Independence 2021

Copyright

Photocopy licence

ISBN-13: 978 1 86168 845 3

Printed in Great Britain

Zenith Print Group

Contents

Introduction

Fertility Issues is Volume 387 in the **issues** series. The aim of the series is to offer current, diverse information about important issues in our world, from a UK perspective.

ABOUT FERTILITY ISSUES

With 1 in 6 couples experiencing problems getting pregnant, fertility is something that not many people think about until they try to conceive. With fertility declining in the UK, we need to make sure that we are aware of the issues that may affect our fertility. This book explores things such as the menstrual cycle, the menopause, alternative ways of having a baby and how lifestyle factors can help or hinder fertility.

OUR SOURCES

Titles in the **issues** series are designed to function as educational resource books, providing a balanced overview of a specific subject.

The information in our books is comprised of facts, articles and opinions from many different sources, including:

♦ Newspaper reports and opinion pieces

♦ Website factsheets

♦ Magazine and journal articles

♦ Statistics and surveys

♦ Government reports

♦ Literature from special interest groups.

A NOTE ON CRITICAL EVALUATION

Because the information reprinted here is from a number of different sources, readers should bear in mind the origin of the text and whether the source is likely to have a particular bias when presenting information (or when conducting their research). It is hoped that, as you read about the many aspects of the issues explored in this book, you will critically evaluate the information presented.

It is important that you decide whether you are being presented with facts or opinions. Does the writer give a biased or unbiased report? If an opinion is being expressed, do you agree with the writer? Is there potential bias to the 'facts' or statistics behind an article?

ASSIGNMENTS

In the back of this book, you will find a selection of assignments designed to help you engage with the articles you have been reading and to explore your own opinions. Some tasks will take longer than others and there is a mixture of design, writing and research-based activities that you can complete alone or in a group.

FURTHER RESEARCH

At the end of each article we have listed its source and a website that you can visit if you would like to conduct your own research. Please remember to critically evaluate any sources that you consult and consider whether the information you are viewing is accurate and unbiased.

Useful Websites

www.bionews.org.uk

www.bupa.co.uk

www.cardiff.ac.uk

www.fertilityed.uk

www.hertsandessexfertility.com

www.independent.co.uk

www.inews.co.uk

www.ivi.uk

www.menopausematters.co.uk

www.metro.co.uk

www.netdoctor.co.uk

www.nhs.uk

www.ons.gov.uk

www.tfp-fertility.com

www.theconversation.com

www.theguardian.com

www.treated.com

A guide to fertility

When are women & men most fertile?

There is only a specific time in each menstrual cycle when it's possible to get pregnant.

This 'fertile window' is once a month, generally close to the time of ovulation when the woman ovulates and releases an egg approximately 2 weeks before the next period is due. Men do not have a 'fertile window' because sperm is continually formed and stored in the testicles, ready to be used at any time.

Graphic 1 shows when pregnancy is most likely to happen in people having sexual intercourse without contraception. Day '0' is the day of ovulation when the egg is released. The pink section in Graphic 1 shows that pregnancy is most likely to happen when sex takes place in the 3 days before ovulation. For example, the chance of pregnancy if people have sex -2 days before ovulation is 26% compared to 1% if they have sex +1 day after ovulation.

Because most women do not know on which day of the month they ovulate, contraception is recommended to avoid pregnancy.

How many months can it take to get pregnant?

If a couple were trying to get pregnant it would be difficult to estimate how long it would take for the woman to get pregnant. Sometimes pregnancy happens quickly but it often takes a few months of trying.

Graphic 2 shows the percentage of men and women having regular unprotected sexual intercourse without contraception who would get pregnant in 1 year, according to their fertility level. By 'regular' we mean having sexual intercourse two to three times per week (National Institute

of Clinical Excellence, 2013). If the couple were fertile, 93% would get pregnant, but if they had a mild fertility problem only 46% would get pregnant. If the couple had serious fertility problems then very few would get pregnant, less than 11%. Examples of fertility problems would be sluggish but forward moving sperm, irregular menstrual periods or one or two blocked fallopian tube(s).

Graphic 2 also shows that even people with mild fertility problems can get pregnant. The National Institute for Health and Care Excellence (NICE) says that if you've been trying to get pregnant for more than 1 year without success then you should talk to your doctor. If you're over 35 or older or think that you or your partner might have a fertility problem then speak to your doctor after 6 months of trying without success.

Graphic 2: Percentage of people who would get pregnant after 1 year of trying

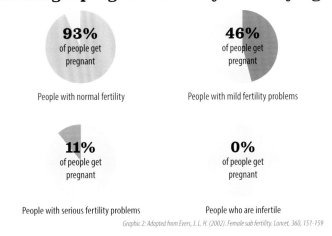

93% of people get pregnant

People with normal fertility

46% of people get pregnant

People with mild fertility problems

11% of people get pregnant

People with serious fertility problems

0% of people get pregnant

People who are infertile

Graphic 2: Adapted from Evers, J. L. H. (2002). Female sub fertility. Lancet, 360, 151-159

Graphic 1: The days in the cycle with the highest chance of getting pregnant

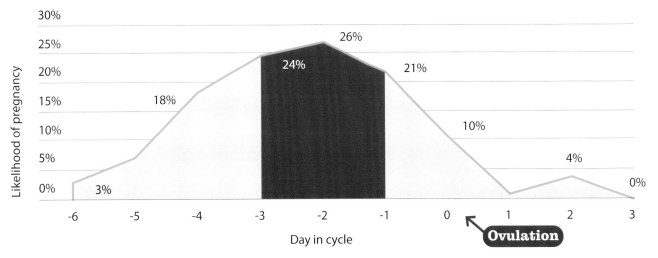

There are ways to help predict ovulation but these methods are not a reliable from of contraception.

Source: Graphic 1: Adapted from Colombo & Masarotto (2000). Daily fecundability: First results from a new database. Demographic Research. Retrieved from http://www.demographic-research.org/volumes/vol3/5/3-5.pdf

Terminology

This guide gives you information about fertility and infertility. To help understand this information we've included an explanation of the main medical terms used.

Ejaculation: Semen is the fluid produced by the male sexual organs to protect and carry sperm. The process of discharging this fluid from the penis is called ejaculation.

Insemination: Treatment that involves directly inserting sperm into a woman's womb

Menstrual cycle: The monthly changes that occur in the female reproductive system (specifically the uterus and ovaries) which make pregnancy possible. The length of the menstrual cycle is calculated as the time from the first day of a woman's period (bleeding) to the day before her next period or bleeding. The average time between two periods for women is about 28 days but in teenagers it could be longer (up to 45 days) and sometimes 2 to 3 months, becoming shorter as the teenager gets older. There are events that occur during the menstrual cycle which are repeated each month. These are: development of the egg (phase 1), release of the egg from one of the ovaries (phase 2), preparation of the uterus for a pregnancy (phase 3), and menstruation or bleeding (phase 4). The next period then happens if there is no pregnancy. Young women should have regular periods within 3 years of the first period occurring. Women could have some spotting in early pregnancy.

Menopause: The menopause is the time when menstrual periods stop permanently, and women are no longer able to have children. For most women this happens at about 51 years. The age a woman will reach menopause will generally be similar to the age at which her mother reached menopause.

Ovulation: is the release of the oocyte (mature egg, sometimes called ovum) from the ovaries, ready for fertilization. Ovulation occurs about two weeks before the next period is due, for example around day 14 of a 28-day cycle or day 21 of a 35-day cycle. The actual day of release could differ between cycles and between women, and is affected by many factors (e.g. lifestyle).

Ovaries: The two oval-shaped organs located in the lower abdomen (right and left side) that produce the female eggs.

Eggs and sperm: Cells that are produced by the ovary (eggs, oocytes, ova) and testicles (sperm) and that combine after sex to produce a pregnancy. Women produce eggs and men produce sperm. A healthy sperm is motile, which means it has the ability to move. This movement is what makes it possible for sperm to reach the egg.

Testicles also called testes or balls: Oval-shaped organs that sit in a sac that hangs behind the penis. A main job of testicles is to make and store sperm.

At what age does fertility begin to decrease?

Girls are born with a fixed number of immature eggs in their ovaries. The number of eggs decreases as women get older. At birth, most girls have about 2 million eggs, at adolescence that number has gone down to about 400, 000, at age 37 there remain about 25,000. By age 51 when women have their menopause they have about 1000 immature eggs but these are not fertile. At every menstrual cycle one of the immature eggs will mature and be released during ovulation. The eggs that are not released die and get re-absorbed into the body. The quality of the eggs also gets poorer as women get older. All other things being equal the number and quality of the woman's eggs determines her fertility.

Graphic 3 shows that on average there is a marked decline in female fertility in the mid-thirties, with lower fertility especially after the age of 35. Women's fertility will continue to decrease every year, whether or not she is healthy and fit because the number and quality of the eggs decreases with age. Even if a woman is not ovulating (for example if she is taking the contraceptive pill, or is pregnant), the number of eggs continues to decline at the same rate. How quick a woman's fertility declines will depend on a combination of genetic and lifestyle (e.g. smoking) factors.

Men are not born with their sperm. Men produce sperm daily. Men's fertility also starts to decline around age 40 to 45. The decrease in fertility is caused by the decrease in the number and quality of the sperm they produce. Men can have fertility problems even if they can still have sex and have an ejaculation.

If you are concerned about your age and your fertility, you may consider having your fertility tested. Fertility tests for men and women are available at pharmacies, online and at fertility clinics. You can discuss your fertility with your doctor.

Graphic 3: Monthly fertility rate by age

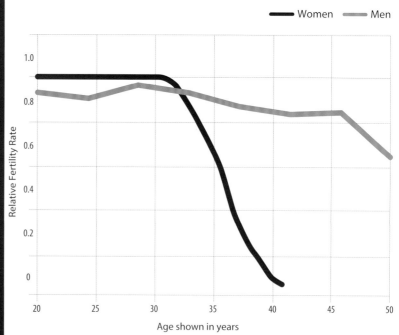

Source: Graphic 3: Reprinted with permission from Trends in Endocrinology and Metabolism, 18, Broekmans, F. J., et al. Female reproductive ageing: current knowledge and future trends, p. 59, 2007, with permission from Elsevier. Male data not in original.
Adapted by permission from BMJ Publishing Group Limited. [Delaying childbearing: effect of age on fecundity and outcome of pregnancy, van Noord-Zaadstra et al., 302, p. 1363, 1991]

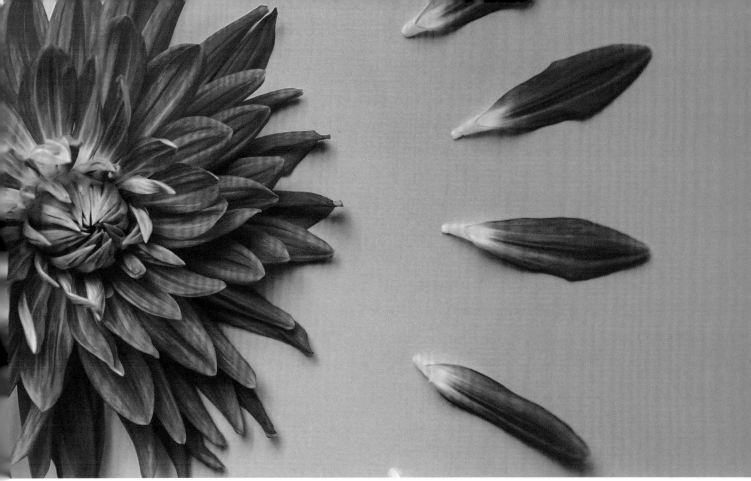

When should you start trying to get pregnant?

Because the fertility of women declines, many women who want children want to know at what age they should try to get pregnant to have a good chance of having the family they want. Researchers have created a chart that may help women (and their partners) make that decision.

To use the chart you need to know:

1. The size of family you would like (e.g. 1, 2, or 3 children)

2. Whether you would be willing to use fertility treatments (e.g. IVF) if you or your partner could not become pregnant naturally

3. Your desired certainty that you will achieve the family size you want (e.g. 50%, 75%, or 90% sure).

Graphic 4 shows when a woman would need to start trying to get pregnant to have the number of children she wanted.

For example, the red numbers show that if a woman wanted to be 90% certain that she would have at least 3 children without ever using fertility treatment, then she would need to start trying for a family at 23. But, she could start aged 36, if she was willing to use fertility treatment and have a lower certainty (50%) of having 3 children (see green numbers). Women (and their partners) can use this chart to decide when to start trying to get pregnant. If you know you have fertility problems that can be overcome with fertility treatment then look at the ages with fertility treatment (with IVF). Such a chart does not yet exist for men.

2017

Graphic 4: Maximum female age at which women should start trying to get pregnant for 1, 2, or 3 children and for a 50%, 75% and 90% chance of reaching the desired family size with and without using fertility treatment

	Chance of meeting family size goal	1 child	2 children	3 children
Without IVF	50%	41 yr	38 yr	35 yr
	75%	37 yr	34 yr	31 yr
	90%	32 yr	27 yr	23 yr
With IVF	50%	42 yr	39 yr	36 yr
	75%	39 yr	35 yr	33 yr
	90%	35 yr	31 yr	28 yr

Source: Graphic 4: Habbema, J. D. F., Eijkemans, M. J. C., Leridon, H., & te Velde, E. R. (2015). Realizing a desired family size: when should couples start? Human Reproduction, 30, 2215-2221. By permission of Oxford University Press.

The above information is reprinted with kind permission from 'A Guide to Fertility' produced by ©Professor Jacky Boivin, Cardiff University 2021

www.fertilityed.uk

www.cardiff.ac.uk

Our complete calendar guide to periods and the menstrual cycle

By Dr. Daniel Atkinson

The menstrual cycle is a fundamental part of life for all women but it is a topic which often goes undiscussed.

Many may have questions relating to the links between conception and the menstrual cycle, but be hesitant to ask their regular GP.

Why are periods sometimes inconsistent? What can affect them? Is there are a time of the month where it is harder or easier to get pregnant?

To help those who may be unsure, below we have supplied a helpful calendar guide to the monthly menstruation cycle, along with some answers to a number of regularly asked questions relating to menstruation and conception.

Menstruation calendar

Day 1

Signified by the first day of your period when you experience a 'bleed'.

This is triggered by a drop in the progesterone hormone when the body recognises that fertilisation of the egg has not occurred. The endometrium must be renewed in preparation for a new egg.

Days 3-7

Bleeding usually stops around this point. A number of eggs in the ovaries begin to mature ready for release at the point of ovulation.

Days 7-14

One egg will continue to develop and reach maturity. The lining of the womb will start to thicken in preparation for ovulation.

Day 14

Around this time, a change in female hormones will cause the mature egg to be propelled out of the ovary to commence its journey.

This is known as ovulation.

Over the next few days the egg will travel down the fallopian tubes eventually meeting the womb.

If you have unprotected sex at this stage a sperm may come into contact and thus fertilise your egg. The combined cells will travel into the womb where they will attach themselves to the thickened endometrium and begin to develop.

Day 25

If the egg has not been fertilised hormone levels will drop and the egg will be broken down. The new period will begin in the next few days.

What is the menstrual cycle?

The menstrual cycle is the term given to the monthly process followed by the female reproductive system.

It covers ovulation, fertility and periods. The length of the cycle is measured from the first day of the period to the day before the next period. For many women this is about 28 days but can vary.

Periods tend to start when someone reaches puberty, typically around the age of twelve, although they can start

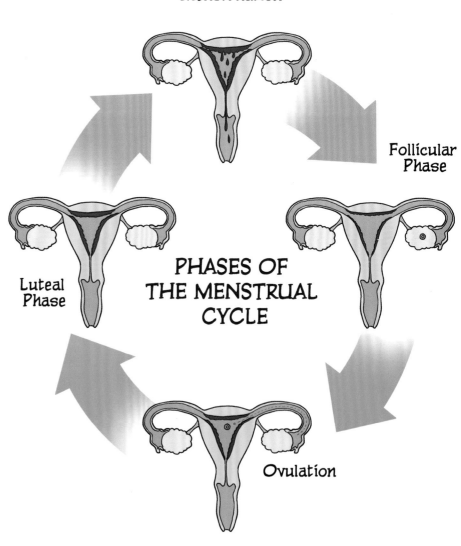

Menstruation

Follicular Phase

PHASES OF THE MENSTRUAL CYCLE

Luteal Phase

Ovulation

earlier or later. The ovaries start to produce female hormones around this time which trigger the different episodes in the cycle.

What is ovulation?

Ovulation refers to the release of a developed egg from the ovaries. For women who follow a regular 28 day cycle this is usually around day 14.

Levels of the oestrogen hormone rise initiating the ovulation process, whilst progesterone thickens the lining of the womb.

During each menstrual cycle a mature egg is released from the ovaries. This is usually just one single egg but occasionally two might develop and be released at the same time. The egg lives for approximately 24 hours during which time it passes into the fallopian tube.

If fertilisation by a sperm cell does not take place, the egg will be broken down in the womb and absorbed by the body.

What are periods?

If pregnancy does not occur at the time of ovulation, the thickened womb lining, also known as the endometrium, must be shed in preparation for the following month's lining.

The endometrium is a mucous membrane made up of cell tissue, which is broken down and passed out along with blood via the cervix and through the vagina. This is known as a period and can cause discomfort and pain while the womb actively breaks down the lining.

Women will experience this to varying extents during their periods, and the flow may be heavy or light and can continue for between three and seven days.

The period flow is usually captured by specially made female sanitary products that come in a range of sizes and styles to suit individual preference. The most commonly used products include tampons, pads and menstrual cups, all of which absorb or capture the menstrual fluid so that it can be disposed of conveniently and hygienically.

What is premenstrual syndrome (PMS)?

Throughout the menstrual cycle, levels of hormones change in the female body; and these fluctuations can sometimes manifest physically in a variety of ways.

In the two weeks prior to the start of a period some women develop symptoms of PMS or premenstrual tension (PMT). These can include but are not solely limited to breast pain, mood swings, being easily irritated, a loss of interest in sex and stomach bloating.

Severe symptoms that prevent the woman from getting on with their daily life may be diagnosed as premenstrual dysphoric disorder (PMDD) which is thought to affect between 2 and 10 percent of menstruating women.

At what stage are you most fertile?

You are most likely to get pregnant around the time of ovulation. Some women notice changes in their body around this time such as breast tenderness, or changes in vaginal discharge and body temperature.

Sperm can live in the fallopian tubes for up to seven days, so it is important to use contraception throughout your cycle if you do not wish to become pregnant.

How long will a person have periods for?

The average ages for starting periods and starting menopause are 12 years and 52 years respectively.

This means that most women will experience periods for around 40 years of their life resulting in close to 480 periods in a lifetime, although this number can obviously vary depending on pregnancies, illnesses and contraception.

Does a 'normal' menstrual cycle exist?

Unfortunately not. Every woman is different and so each cycle can vary in length and flow. The average length of a menstrual cycle is 28 days but this does absolutely not mean that women whose cycles are longer or shorter are 'abnormal'.

The majority of women will lose between 30-40 millilitres of blood during a menstrual bleed but these numbers can increase. Consistent periods where over 60 millilitres of blood is lost may be diagnosed as menorrhagia or heavy periods. There are treatments available to help ease the symptoms of menorrhagia.

What can affect a regular menstruation cycle?

Most women will get to know their own menstrual cycle but there are things that might change or alter it in some way.

The regularity of periods can be affected by stress, sudden changes in weight, diet, medication, health conditions such as polycystic ovary syndrome (PCOS) and of course pregnancy. Your period may be lighter or heavier, occur less frequently or disappear entirely, known clinically as amenorrhoea.

If you have concerns about changes in your menstrual cycle you should speak to your doctor.

Can you have sex during your period?

Yes, however there may be an increased risk of contracting or transmitting sexually transmitted infections (STIs) at this time, so practising safe sex (with a barrier contraceptive) is important. Sex during the menstrual bleed can also be uncomfortable because the cervix may be in a different position to what it is usually.

1 October 2020

Five ages of female fertility

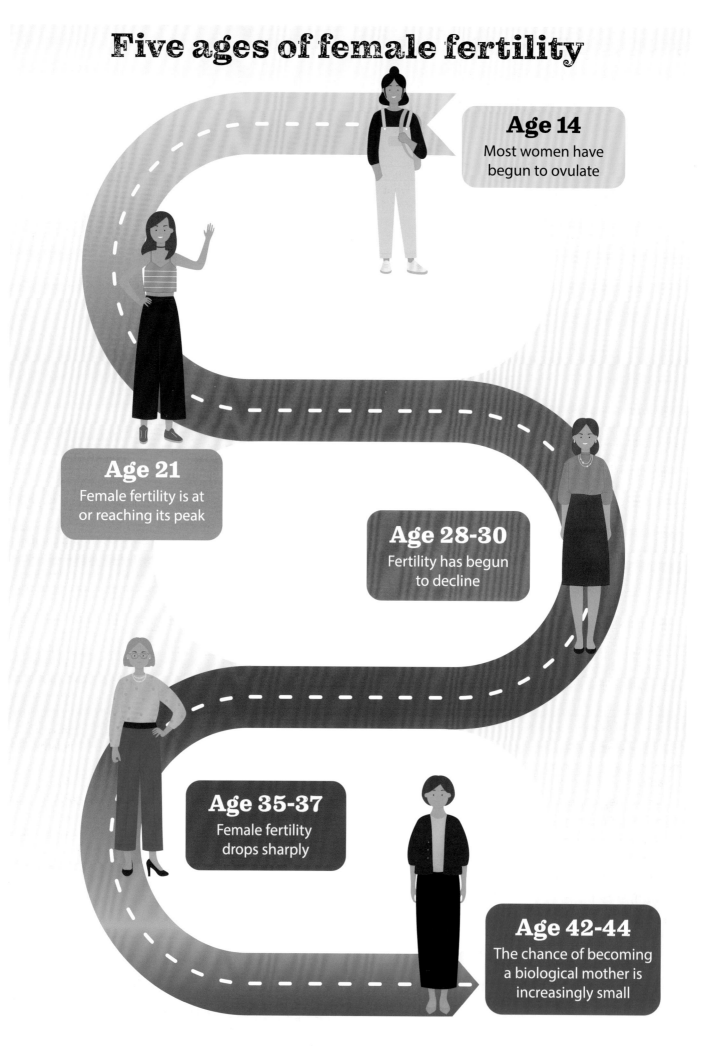

Age 14
Most women have begun to ovulate

Age 21
Female fertility is at or reaching its peak

Age 28-30
Fertility has begun to decline

Age 35-37
Female fertility drops sharply

Age 42-44
The chance of becoming a biological mother is increasingly small

What is the perimenopause?

By Dr Samantha Wild, Clinical Lead for Women's Health and Bupa GP

Often when people talk about 'going through the menopause' they're actually talking about the perimenopause. The perimenopause is when your hormone levels start to change, but before your periods stop for good. It can cause a wide range of symptoms, both physically and mentally. Here I'll talk about what the perimenopause is, ways to cope with it and how to look after your body as it changes.

What triggers the perimenopause?

The perimenopause is a natural stage of life that occurs as you age. In most people it will happen naturally between the ages of 45 and 60, and last for a few months to several years. Even a decade or more. During the perimenopause, your hormone levels change and your ovaries start to produce fewer eggs. Once you haven't had a period for 12 months or more, you've officially reached the menopause.

Some people start experiencing the perimenopause before they are 40. This can be as a result of medical treatments, such as surgery to remove the ovaries, but sometimes there's no cause. If you think you're experiencing the perimenopause before you're 40 then you must speak to your doctor.

What are the signs of the perimenopause?

The symptoms of the perimenopause are caused by the hormonal changes happening in your body. Some people won't have any symptoms, but most will. For some people symptoms can be very severe and affect their daily lives. Everybody's experience will vary, but physical symptoms commonly include:

- changes in your menstrual cycle
- hot flushes and night sweats
- headaches
- dizziness
- vaginal dryness
- incontinence and bladder problems
- weight gain
- joint and muscle pain
- difficulty sleeping

There are also other symptoms of the perimenopause that can affect your feelings and mental health. These include:

- feeling depressed
- experiencing mood swings
- problems with memory and concentration – sometimes called 'brain fog'
- a loss of interest in sex

Managing symptoms of the perimenopause

Just because the perimenopause is a natural process, it doesn't mean that it's always easy to cope with. If you're experiencing symptoms, there are some things that you can do that may help.

- Avoid alcohol and caffeine if they seem to trigger your hot flushes, or if you're having trouble sleeping.

- Use moisturisers and lubricants to help with vaginal dryness.
- If you smoke, try to give up as smoking can increase hot flushes.
- Do things that reduce your stress, such as practising yoga and mindfulness.
- Try to get enough sleep.
- Eat a healthy balanced diet and take part in regular exercise to help manage your weight and give you more energy.

There are also treatments that your doctor can prescribe if you need some support to improve your quality of life. These include:

- hormones, also known as hormone replacement therapy (HRT)
- medicines to ease specific symptoms
- help with your mental health, such as cognitive behavioural therapy (CBT)

You don't need to wait for your periods to stop before speaking to your doctor.

Can I still get pregnant?

Pregnancy is still possible if you're experiencing the perimenopause. However, it's much less likely because you're not ovulating as frequently.

If you don't want to become pregnant, you should continue using contraception until your doctor says it's safe to stop. The right contraceptive for you depends on your age, symptoms and needs, so talk to your doctor about your options.

Preparing for the menopause

Experiencing the perimenopause is a signal that your body is changing. After the menopause you're more likely to develop heart disease and osteoporosis than you were before. The good news is that there are some things you can do to help support your health.

- Eat a heart healthy diet, with at least five portions of fruit and vegetables a day, plenty of fibre, and healthy fats from fish, nuts and seeds.
- Include two to three portions of calcium-rich foods, such as milk, cheese and yoghurt in your daily diet to help support your bones.
- Consider taking a daily supplement of 10 micrograms of vitamin D to help support your bone health.
- Do some moderate exercise for half an hour, five days a week, including strength exercises on two days a week or more.

25 August 2020

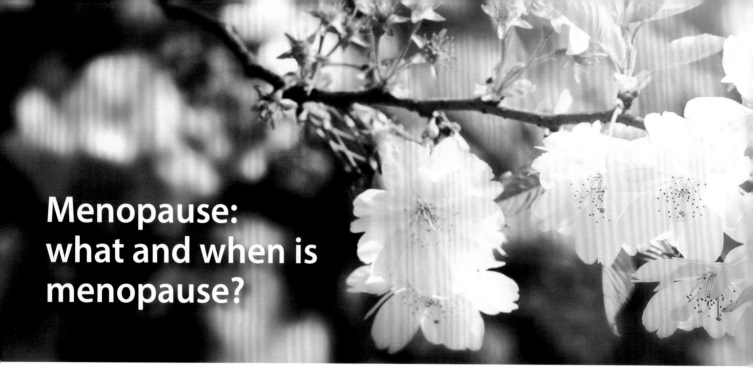

Menopause: what and when is menopause?

Menopause- what happens?

All women will experience the menopause. Natural menopause takes place when the ovaries become unable to produce the hormones estrogen and progesterone. Menopause can also occur when the ovaries are damaged by specific treatment such as chemotherapy or radiotherapy, or when the ovaries are removed, often at the time of a hysterectomy. Ovaries naturally fail to produce estrogen and progesterone when they have few remaining egg cells; the maximum number of egg cells in the ovaries is present before birth, with a reduced number already at birth, gradual reduction from puberty, and a rapid decline from 40 onwards. With less egg cells, the ovaries become less able to respond to hormones from the pituitary gland in the brain: follicle stimulating hormone (FSH) and luteinising hormone (LH) and less estrogen is produced. Levels of FSH and LH subsequently rise and a measurement of FSH is sometimes used to diagnose menopause. The resulting low, and changing levels of ovarian hormones, particularly estrogen, are thought to be the cause of menopausal symptoms and later consequences in many women.

The term **climacteric** refers to the time in which the hormone levels are changing, up to the periods stopping; reducing and changing hormone levels can cause early menopausal symptoms. At this stage, there may still be enough hormones produced to stimulate the lining of the womb (endometrium) to produce monthly periods (menstruation).

Menopause means the last menstrual period. Periods stop because the low levels of estrogen and progesterone do not stimulate the lining of the womb (endometrium) in the normal cycle. Hormone levels can fluctuate for several years before eventually becoming so low that the endometrium stays thin and does not bleed.

Perimenopause is the stage from the beginning of menopausal symptoms to the postmenopause.

Postmenopause is the time following the last period, and is usually defined as more than 12 months with no periods in someone with intact ovaries, or immediately following surgery if the ovaries have been removed.

Menopause - when?

The average age of the natural menopause is 51 years, but can occur much earlier or later. Menopause occurring before the age of 45 is called early menopause and before the age of 40 is premature menopause.

Generally, women having an early or premature menopause are advised to take HRT until approximately the average age of the menopause, for both symptom control and bone protective effect.

Late menopause may also occur but by the age of 54, 80% of women will have stopped having periods.

Menopause symptoms

Why do menopausal symptoms occur and what can we do about them?

Menopausal symptoms, which affect about 70% of women, are believed to be due to the changing hormone levels, particularly estrogen, but many factors such as diet and exercise, lifestyle and other medication can influence the symptoms. Therefore, for some people, life-style factors such as reducing/stopping smoking, reducing alcohol intake, reducing caffeine intake, reducing stress, eating healthily and taking regular exercise can considerably help the symptoms of menopause. For others, HRT can be very beneficial, and indeed menopausal symptom control is the main indication for using HRT. If HRT is taken for symptom relief only, a trial period of stopping HRT is recommended every 2 years or so to assess whether or not treatment is still required. If, on stopping HRT, it's found that menopause symptoms recur then treatment can be restarted if it is felt that the benefits outweigh the risks. Alternative therapies may also be considered for menopause symptom control.

When do menopausal symptoms begin?

Many women notice early symptoms while still having periods, when the hormone production is declining very gradually. This stage of gradually falling and fluctuating hormone levels is often called the 'climacteric' or the 'change' and often begins in the 4th decade and can last for

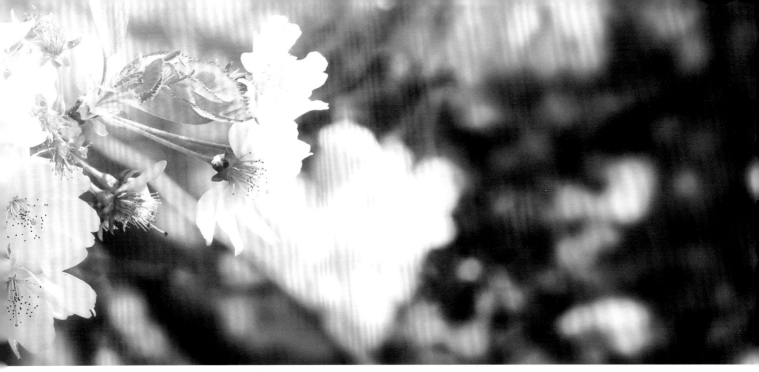

several years. Because ovarian function fluctuates, women may experience menopause symptoms intermittently. Some women experience an early, or premature menopause following which, symptoms may occur immediately, depending on the cause. Immediate onset of menopause symptoms often follows a surgical menopause. The duration of 'early' symptoms is very variable from a few months to many years and the severity varies between individuals.

Early menopause symptoms

Early menopause symptoms include physical, sexual and psychological problems.

Physical symptoms include:

- Hot flushes
- Night sweats
- Palpitations
- Insomnia
- Joint aches
- Headaches

The hot flush, or flash, is well known as the classic menopausal symptom and affects 60–85% of menopausal women. Hot flushes and sweats are called vasomotor symptoms and vary immensely in both their severity and duration; for many women, they occur occasionally and do not cause much distress, but for about 20% they can be severe and can cause significant interference with work, sleep and quality of life. Women are affected by vasomotor symptoms on average for about 2 years but, for about 10%, symptoms can continue for more than 15 years. Hot flushes usually last 3–5 minutes and are thought to be caused by a change in the temperature-controlling part of the brain. Normally, there is a daily pattern of rises and falls in your body temperature, being lowest at about 3am and highest in the early evening. These small changes are not normally noticed, but a menopausal woman may flush with every temperature rise, whether these are normal changes or not – for example, moving between areas of different temperature or having a hot drink – because of a change in the setting of the temperature control centre in your brain; your body thinks

that it is overheating even when it isn't. To try to cool your body down, a variety of chemical reactions cause the blood vessels in the skin to open up, giving the sensation of a rush of heat, and sweat glands release sweat to dissipate heat. It is believed that the changes in various hormone levels that occur around the time of the menopause lead to the change in the setting of the temperature control centre, but the exact underlying mechanism is still unclear. Other factors that can also cause flushes include being overweight, alcohol, excess caffeine, spicy foods, monosodium glutamate and some medications. Eating a healthy diet and losing weight if necessary can be helpful. Other simple measures that can help include:

- wearing cotton clothing rather than man-made fibres
- wearing loose thin layers of clothing rather than thick tight-fitting clothes
- keeping your bedroom temperature fairly cool at night – either leave a door or window open or consider a fan (partner permitting of course!).

Flushes affect every woman differently and, for many, no specific treatments will be required. When flushes are embarrassing, disruptive and affecting your quality of life, then help is available and your doctor will give you an individualised treatment plan – we are all unique! Headaches, palpitations (sensation of heart racing) and dizziness can be associated with vasomotor symptoms. Excess caffeine can worsen palpitations, so take coffee, tea and caffeinated soft drinks in moderation.

Insomnia (sleeplessness) or disturbed sleep (leading to tiredness and fatigue), may be partly due to the night sweats, control of which can lead to an improved sleep pattern.

Joint aches commonly occur, often affecting neck, wrists, and shoulders but recognition of their possible association to menopause is often lacking. Visit our Forum for more information on menopausal joint aches and to find out how others have coped.

Psychological menopause symptoms such as mood swings, irritability, anxiety, difficulty concentrating, difficulty coping and forgetfulness may be related to hormonal changes, either directly or indirectly, e.g. due to sleep disturbance. However, other life events such as worry over elderly relatives, teenage children, and pressures from work commonly occur around the time of menopause and may contribute to such 'symptoms'.

Sexual Problems may be caused by vaginal dryness due to low estrogen levels, resulting in discomfort during intercourse. Effective treatments are available. As both men and women get older, interest in sex may decrease but this particularly affects women. Treatment of other menopausal symptoms may indirectly improve libido by improving feelings of well-being and energy levels, e.g. by improving sleep through control of night sweats, but restoring hormone levels can also improve sensation. Relationship problems have an obvious effect on libido, so hormonal treatment may not always be the 'magic' solution!

Later menopause symptoms

Later menopause symptoms are due to the effects of estrogen deficiency on the bladder and vagina and include:

♦ Passing urine more often by day and/or by night

♦ Discomfort on passing urine

♦ Urine infection

♦ Leakage of urine

♦ Vaginal dryness, discomfort, discharge, burning and itching

Although bladder and vaginal symptoms can occur in the early stages of the menopause, they most often occur a few years after the last period, or a few years after stopping HRT.

Vaginal and bladder symptoms are very common and can cause significant distress yet are often under-reported and under-treated. Women are frequently too embarrassed to discuss these problems. Very effective treatments are available and should be discussed. For vaginal dryness, non-hormonal vaginal moisturisers may be used. For bladder and vaginal symptoms, and to treat the underlying cause, ie lack of estrogen, local vaginal estrogen (tablet, cream, pessary or ring) can be very helpful. Low dose, vaginal estrogen can be used when systemic estrogen is inappropriate and can be continued in the long-term without any known adverse effects. Vaginal estrogen may be required in addition to systemic HRT since in some women, the systemic HRT, although helping symptoms such as flushes, may not be sufficiently helpful for vaginal symptoms.

Other menopause symptoms

Other later menopause symptoms include effects from changes in collagen production, a protein in skin, hair, nails and tendons. As its production is affected by falling estrogen levels, the skin may become dryer, thinner, less elastic, more prone to bruising, and skin itching may occur. Occasionally, a 'crawling' sensation may be experienced but it is unclear whether this is due to skin changes or changes in the peripheral nerves. Skin symptoms often respond to estrogen replacement, but some women have developed skin itch when taking HRT. In this situation, a change in type or route of HRT may help.

Hair thinning, dryness and the growth of unwanted hair can be explained by the lack of estrogen and the relative excess of androgens in the menopause (the adrenal glands and the ovaries continue to produce some androgens including testosterone, the effect of which is no longer overridden by estrogen). However, hair loss may be more dependent on age rather than hormone related and response to HRT is unclear. Thyroid disease and iron deficiency can also cause hair loss and should be considered, particularly if there are other signs.

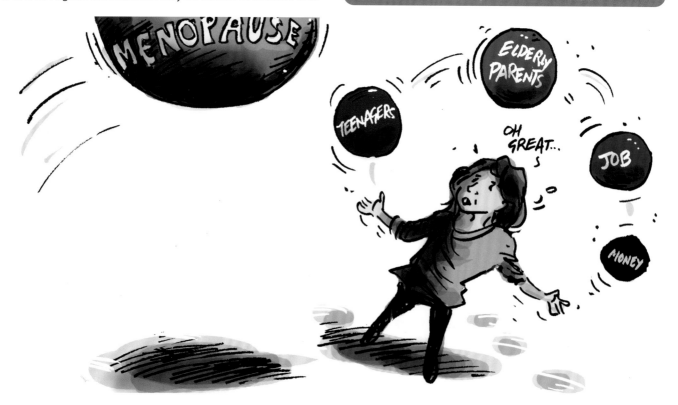

Births in England and Wales: 2019

An extract.

Main points

♦ There were 640,370 live births in England and Wales in 2019, a decrease of 2.5% since 2018 and a 12.2% decrease since the most recent peak in 2012.

♦ The total fertility rate (TFR) for England and Wales decreased from 1.70 children per woman in 2018 to 1.65 children per woman in 2019; this is lower than all previous years except 2000, 2001 and 2002.

♦ The TFR for Wales was the lowest since records began in 1982 at 1.54 children per woman.

♦ Fertility rates for women in age groups under 30 years were at the lowest level since records began in 1938.

♦ Fertility rates decreased in all age groups except for women aged 40 years and over, among whom the rate increased to 16.5 births per 1,000 women.

♦ The stillbirth rate for England fell to a record low for the third consecutive year to 3.8 stillbirths per 1,000 total births, while the stillbirth rate for Wales increased from 4.4 to 4.6 stillbirths per 1,000 total births in 2019.

Statistician's comment

'The story of births in England and Wales in 2019 is one of decreases and record lows, with the total number of births continuing the fall we've seen in recent years. Wales had the lowest fertility rate since our records began and England's is nearing its record low.

David Corps, Vital Statistics Outputs Branch, Office for National Statistics

Number of births and fertility rates

The number of live births in England and Wales decreased for the fourth consecutive year. In 2019, there were 640,370 live births; this is a 2.5% decrease from 657,076 live births in 2018 and the fewest since 2004.

The total fertility rate (TFR) was lower in 2019 than in all previous years except 2000, 2001 and 2002. The TFR accounts for the size and age structure of the female population of childbearing age and therefore provides a better measure of trends than simply looking at the number of live births.

In 2019, the TFR in England and Wales fell to 1.65 children per woman, a 2.9% decrease from 2018. TFRs have been decreasing year on year since 2013 (Figure 1). The TFR provides a timely measure of fertility levels and can be affected by changes in the timing of childbearing, completed family size and the population structure.

Possible reasons for the decrease in TFRs in recent years could be:

♦ improved access to contraception

♦ the reduction in mortality rates of children aged under 5 years, resulting in women having fewer babies

♦ lower levels of fertility, or difficulties conceiving because of postponement in childbearing

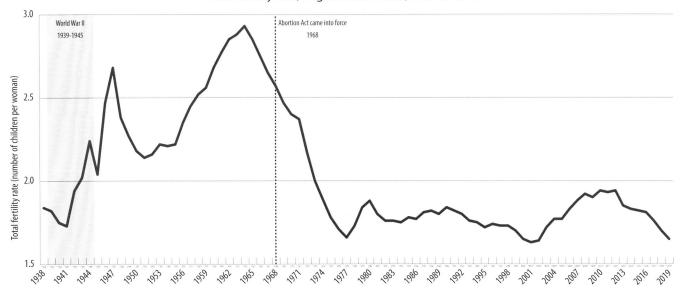

Figure 1: The total fertility rate decreased for the seventh consecutive year
Total fertility rate, England and Wales, 1938 to 2019

Notes:

1. Based on live births occurring in each calendar year, plus a very small number of late registrations from the previous year.

2. The total fertility rate is the average number of live children that a group of women would bear if they experienced the age-specific fertility rates of the calendar year throughout their childbearing lifespan.

Source: Office for National Statistics – Births in England and Wales

Figure 2: Fertility rates for women aged under 30 years have generally been decreasing since 2013

Age-specific fertility rates, England and Wales, 1938 to 2019

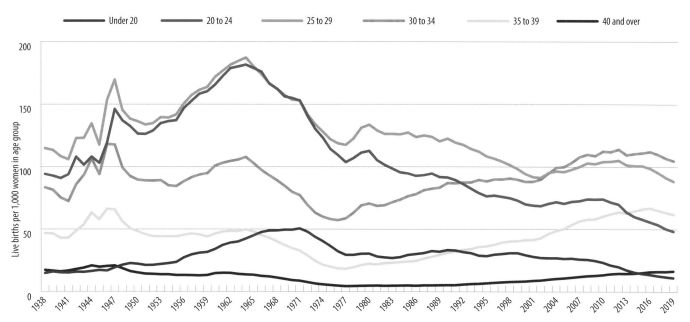

Notes:

1. Based on live births occurring in each calendar year, plus a very small number of late registrations from the previous year.
2. The rates for women aged under 20 years and aged 40 years and over are based on the female population aged 15 to 19 years and 40 to 44 years respectively.
3. Age-specific fertility rates for 1981 are based on a 10% sample because of the late submission of some birth registrations resulting from a registrars' strike.
4. The population estimates used to calculate fertility rates from 1938 to 1980 are rounded to the nearest hundred and are therefore of a slightly lower level of accuracy than the fertility rates for 1981 onwards.

Source: Office for National Statistics – Births in England and Wales

Fertility rates by age of mother

The standardised mean age of mother at childbirth was 30.7 years and has been gradually increasing since 1973 when it was 26.4 years. This trend is replicated in age-specific fertility rates (ASFRs) where, for the fifth consecutive year, the fertility rate for women aged under 20 years (11.2) was lower than the rate for women aged 40 years and over (16.5); this is a pattern last recorded in 1947. Fertility rates for women aged over 40 years have been steadily increasing since 1978 (Figure 2).

In 2019, the ASFRs in each age group for women aged under 30 years were at their lowest levels since records began in 1938. Fertility rates for women in the age groups under 30 years have generally been decreasing each year since 2013 (Figure 2).

These trends suggest women are progressively delaying childbearing to older ages. Reasons for women delaying having children until later in life could include:

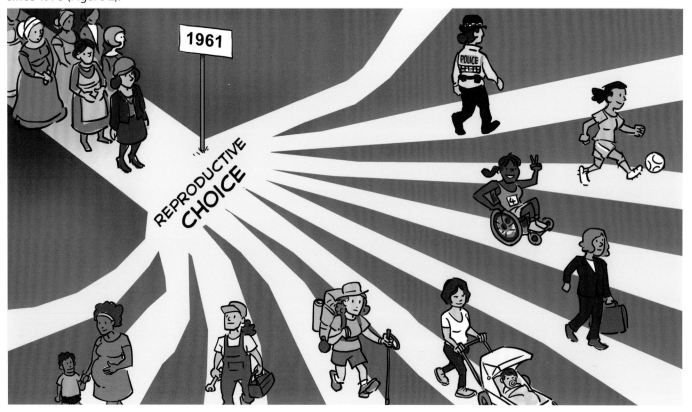

12

Figure 4: Between 2017 and 2018 total fertility rates (TFRs) decreased in the majority of local authorities

Total fertility rates by local authority district, England and Wales, 2001 to 2018

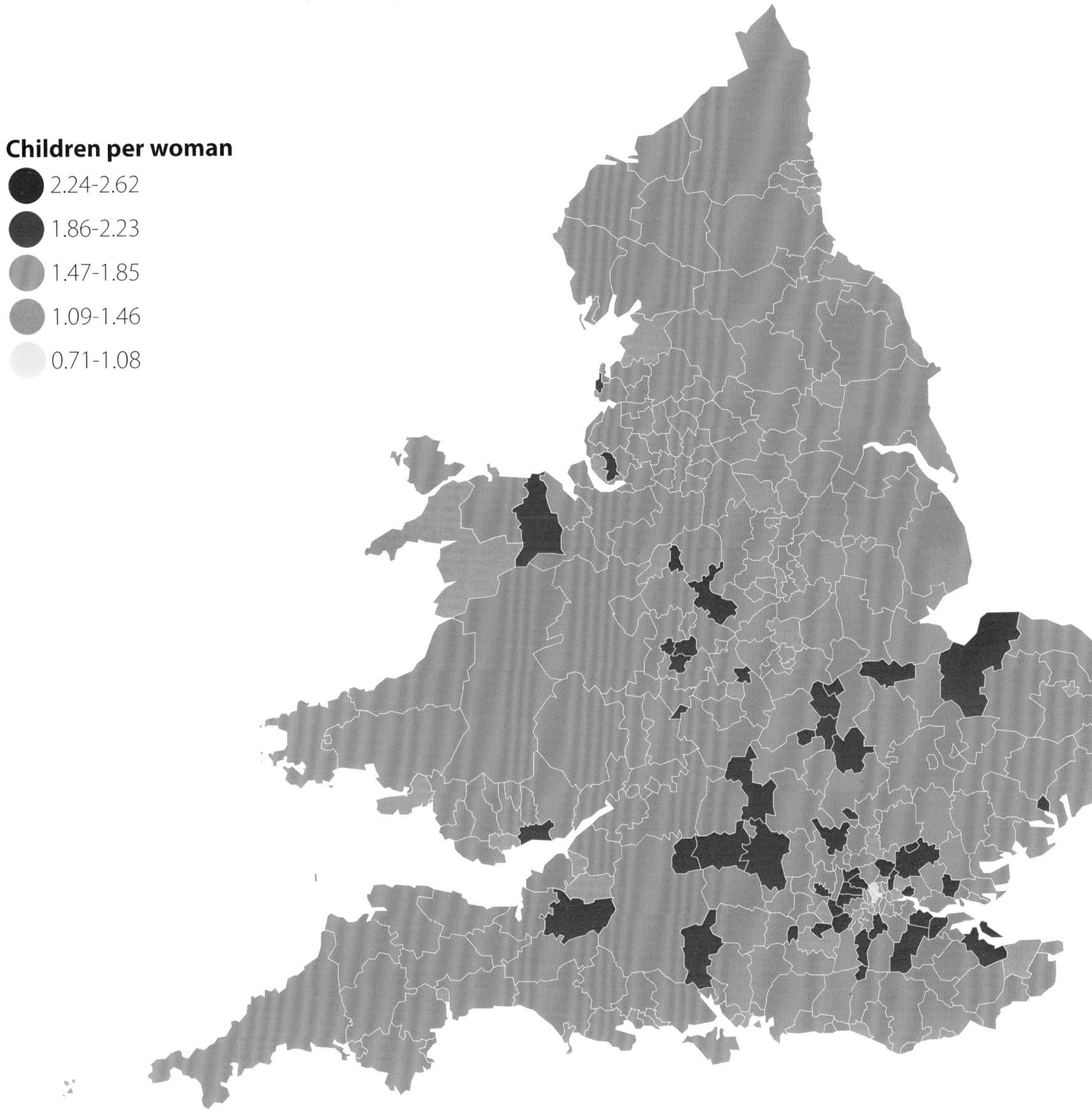

Children per woman

- 2.24-2.62
- 1.86-2.23
- 1.47-1.85
- 1.09-1.46
- 0.71-1.08

Notes:

1. The total fertility rate is the average number of live children that a group of women would bear if they experienced the age-specific fertility rates of the calendar year throughout their childbearing lifespan.

2. The Isles of Scilly has been combined with Cornwall for all years because of the very small number of births in this area.

3. Figures are based on mothers' usual area of residence, based on boundaries as of May 2020.

Source: Office for National Statistics – Births in England and Wales

- greater participation in higher education

- delaying marriage and/or partnership formation

- wanting to have a longer working career before starting a family

- labour market uncertainty and the threat of unemployment

Fertility rates by geographic area

The total fertility rate (TFR) in England was 1.66 children per woman in 2019, a decrease of 2.4% compared with 2018. The TFR in Wales was the lowest since records began in 1982 at 1.54 children per woman, a 5.5% decrease from the previous year.

Across all English regions, the TFR decreased compared with 2018. The regions with the highest and lowest TFRs remained the same as 2018, with the East being the highest at 1.77 children per woman and the North East the lowest with 1.52 children per woman.

The map (Figure 4) shows the changes in TFRs from 2001 to 2018 across England and Wales. In 2019, the local authorities with both the lowest and highest TFR were in London.

When we look at fertility rates in even smaller areas, like in Figure 4, it is important to consider the numbers involved. In some local authorities, the total childbearing population is small, so if there is a small change in the number of live births in these areas, there can be large changes in the TFRs. Other variations can be a result of differences in the characteristics of the population living in each area such as social, economic and cultural differences.

22 July 2020

Top 10 fertility myths now busted

There are many misconceptions around infertility and fertility treatments in general and we've decided to explain why some of these mislead people or couples trying to conceive.

By Dr Jyoti Taneja, Consultant Gynaecology & Reproductive Medicine

1: Infertility is a female problem – myth busted

Infertility is the inability of a person to reproduce by natural means and can occur in both men and women.

Heterosexual couples may struggle to conceive naturally either due to fertility problems that may occur in one partner or even both. Heterosexual couples can also experience unexplained infertility which means that the available examinations and tests conducted may not explain what causes the infertility.

LGBTQ couples or single people can also struggle with fertility. Most commonly called situational infertility, because biologically they cannot have a child. In other words, they may need fertility treatments, like insemination with a sperm donor, or treatment using donor gametes (donor eggs/donor sperm/donor embryo) or the help of a surrogate to carry the pregnancy.

In cases of same sex female relationship they may face medical causes of infertility on top of situational infertility. It may be that one or both female partners are unable to conceive because they have an underlying fertility problem and may require fertility drugs or other treatments in addition to needing a sperm donor.

2: Male ejaculation equals fertility – myth busted

Men with male infertility have no visible or obvious signs that something is wrong.

A healthy erectile function and normal ejaculation does not guarantee that your sperm is functionally normal. Some men have 100% antibodies, which may be the reason no fertilization with an egg happens despite normal sperm count numbers.

It's a myth that if a man's fertility is compromised, then his sexual performance will also always be affected, as some will not have any sexual problems.

Abnormalities with sperm count, shape, and movement are not always the cause of male infertility. You can't tell there is a problem with your sperm only by looking at semen. The functionality of sperm can be tested using some special tests like DNA fragmentation tests or Hyaluronan Binding Assay (HBA analysis), which give more information on the functional analysis.

Semen is also made up of fluids and mucus rich in sugars, amino acids, hormones, and minerals, all intended to support the sperm cells and help keep them alive outside of the man's body, and if any of these parameters are not optimal, this may also contribute to no fertilization.

3: Age doesn't matter, there's always IVF – myth busted

There is a common misconception that if age-related infertility does strike, you can always do IVF. This is far from the truth, because just as your natural fertility declines with age, your odds for success with IVF treatment also decline with age.

For women less than 35 years of age, who have normal ovarian reserve, 30-35% percent of IVF cycles will lead to the

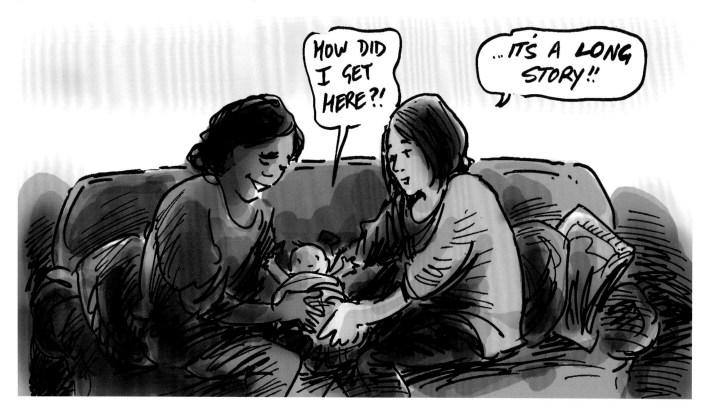

livebirth of a baby. For women aged 38 to 40, the success rate drops to almost half. Very few women aged 43 to 44, will have a live birth using their own eggs.

Women may opt to consider donor egg treatment if age-related infertility stands in the way of parenthood, but treatment using donor eggs may not always guarantee success.

4: Clomid can help anyone get pregnant faster – myth busted

Clomiphene citrate (Clomid) is an anti-estrogen drug to stimulate ovulation in women with irregular or absent ovulation. But if you don't have any of these problems, ovulation induction may not help. In fact, Clomid reduces the fertile quality of cervical mucus. It makes cervical fluids stickier and less abundant. Cervical mucus helps sperm survive and swim from the cervix up into the reproductive system. There are several other drugs used for ovulation induction viz Tamoxifen, Letrozole.

If you don't have problems that indicate ovulation induction, then it may not improve your fertility.

5: Egg reserve can reduce or finish if many eggs are collected at egg collection – myth busted

In a natural cycle, depending on ovarian reserve, women ovulate with mostly 1 or 2 eggs, and have some others which wither away in that month as not all of these are suitable for ovulation due to natural hormone levels. In treatment cycles medication helps stimulate most of those recruited follicles in that month to get them ready for egg collection. In the following month there will be newer follicles recruited again depending on ovarian reserve.

6: IVF frequently leads to higher-order pregnancies – myth busted

Out of all the available types of fertility treatments, IVF is the least likely to lead to a higher-order pregnancy with triplets, quadruplets or more. With IVF treatment, embryos are transferred back to the uterus, and most reproductive specialists will transfer one and in some circumstances not more than two embryos at a time. In fact, elective single embryo transfer is becoming more popular. This is the safe option recommended to most patients to have a healthy, singleton pregnancy. There is always still a minuscule risk of identical twins despite single embryo transfer.

7: After embryo transfer, the embryo slips out if you stand up quickly – myth busted

This is a common concern in women having an embryo transfer that mobilizing quickly or going to the toilet will make the embryo slip out, which is not true as the embryo is microscopic in the folds of endometrium, and no amount of movement will make it slip out.

Another common query amongst women after embryo transfer is whether they should just lie in bed. In fact moving

about is recommended for good circulation and vital for minimizing risks of clots. Gentle walks in the fresh air are good for healthy pregnancy.

8: After IVF you cannot have an Ectopic pregnancy – myth busted

Putting the embryo back in the uterus does not mean it cannot transport back further and implant in any other ectopic area like the fallopian tubes, cervix, ovary or cornual area of uterus: which is not conducive to a healthy pregnancy and may entail surgical management in some cases. This is higher where there is underlying disease pathology in these ectopic areas.

9: If you already have a child, you don't need to worry about fertility – myth busted

Secondary infertility is when a couple has difficulty getting pregnant after they have conceived a child naturally in the past. Unfortunately, a previous successful pregnancy doesn't guarantee fertility success in future.

Changes come with time and age in fertility. It could be related to an underlying new medical or gynaecological condition or a fertility condition that always existed and got worse, and while it didn't prevent pregnancy in the past, now it has become a problem.

Occasionally a previous pregnancy could cause a fertility problem in cases of surgical complications or infections after childbirth.

10: IVF treatment will definitely get you pregnant – myth busted

This simply isn't true. Success after any form of fertility treatment is not guaranteed.

With treatments, you could move to using an egg donor, sperm donor, embryo donor or a surrogate and may still not be successful. This process can include a tremendous amount of time, emotions and financial cost.

Moving on is an option everyone should be able to take without any guilt that the next cycle could have been the one. Yes, maybe it could have been but it also might not have, and you are only doing your best in your situation.

Infertility and fertility treatments can be overwhelming as there is a lot of misleading information. How can you know what's right in your case? Talk to a fertility specialist doctor for clarifications on your personal situation, medical diagnosis and treatment options.

26 February 2019

Male fertility facts you need to know in your 20's

If you see children in your future, here's some information that you need to know…

Infertility impacts men, as much as women

Over a third of all fertility problems are due to the male factor (and sperm) in conceiving. This shows you how common it is.

Age and male fertility

As you get older, your fertility does decline. Ageing impacts the quality and quantity of sperm. Many however go on to successfully conceive later in life.

When does male fertility drop off?

Although the decline in fertility is less dramatic for men, the gradual decline starts in the late 20s.

Signs of male infertility and male infertility symptoms

Not all men experience signs and symptoms of infertility. Often, many men go through their 20's completely unaware of any issues with their fertility and most will only become aware of their fertility when they are trying to conceive. Male Infertility

What are the most common reasons for male fertility issues?

Defects in your reproductive system, low hormone levels, childhood and current illnesses, or medications might harm sperm production. Lifestyle factors such as high BMI, smoking, excessive consumption of alcohol and recreational drugs can also affect sperm.

Reduced sperm count, motility and abnormal sperm shape are the common abnormalities found in the sperm.

Is male fertility treatable?

Yes, many treatments exist to help men who are trying to conceive.

How do I establish my fertility?

In order to establish your fertility and the right treatment for you, consultation with a fertility specialist, physical examination and diagnostic testing are needed. Semen analysis is a routine laboratory test that helps to identify the quality and quantity of the sperm. The quality of your sperm tells much about your ability to start a pregnancy.

Lifestyle and male fertility

Your lifestyle can impact your fertility and sperm quality. Key things to watch in your 20's include your diet and BMI, smoking and substance use, as well as alcohol consumption, STI's and medication. If you have a medical condition that can impact your fertility, then your GP or consultant will be able to give you further information.

Your chances of conceiving

Everybody's chances of conceiving are different because everybody is different. Sometimes it takes longer for a couple to conceive, other times it does not. Typically, a healthy young couple's chances of conceiving in year one is around 80%. Of those that do not conceive in year one, half will naturally conceive in year two.

A rule of thumb to follow is that as a couple, if you have been trying to conceive for over a year and you are concerned, then do make an appointment to see a fertility specialist. If you are part of an older couple or you are aware of a medical condition/lifestyle factor that could be impacting your fertility, then we would recommend that you seek out a fertility specialist sooner, rather than later.

Treatable male fertility issues

Fertility specialists are able to perform individualised tests and consultations to establish the best treatment for you. Common sperm abnormalities that could be overcome by fertility treatment include:

♦ No sperm production

♦ Low sperm count Treatable Male Fertility Issues

♦ Low sperm motility

♦ Past vasectomy

♦ Irregular sperm shape and structure

♦ Hormone imbalance

Is IVF the answer for male infertility?

Not necessarily, many treatments are available to help treat male infertility. A fertility specialist will help you to increase your chances of success by selecting the best treatment for you. Examples of other common male fertility treatments include Intracytoplasmic Sperm Injection (ICSI), Surgical sperm retrieval and sperm donation.

If you have questions or concerns about male fertility, remember you are not alone and there are people who can help.

www.tfp-fertility.com

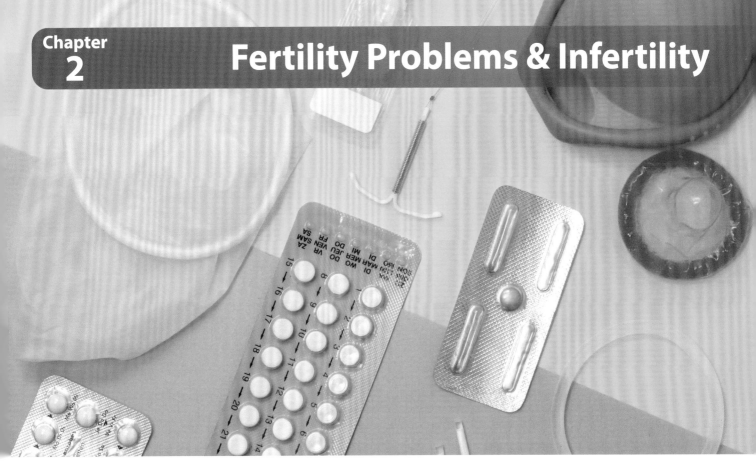

Can birth control cause fertility problems?

By Cesar Diaz-Garcia, MD PhD Assoc Prof

Effective birth control is one of the transformative medical advances that has allowed generations of women to take control of their own destinies. It's easy to forget that since the pill was introduced in the UK in 1961, we have been at liberty to enjoy a level of personal freedom that our grandmothers never knew. **Absolutely, birth control pills can cause infertility**: that is what they are designed for! But of course that type of elective, temporary protection from involuntary pregnancy is not what we think of as infertility.

Just as women want reliable contraception at certain times, we also need reassurance that, when the time comes to try for pregnancy, there won't be a backlash from previous contraception. So can birth control cause infertility? The good news is that it doesn't, but different types of birth control can cause a small fertility delay.

Types of birth control and infertility

We all know that if you stop using a barrier method like condoms or a diaphragm, you can get pregnant the moment you stop using them. Most people's doubts and concerns focus on the longer term effects of hormonal contraceptives, whether these are a pill, an implant or an injection. Some methods do carry a risk of having to wait a few months for fertility to return to square one. This is probably what gives rise to the myth that birth control pills can cause infertility. How do the main birth control methods compare?

♦ **The combination pill.** This is one that contains both progesterone and oestrogen. It works by preventing ovulation as well as thickening the mucus at the neck of the womb and thinning the lining avoiding the ovulation and making the implantation less likely. According to the NHS, it is 99% effective when taken correctly, which is what makes it rightly very popular. When you stop taking it, your cycles should be back to normality. Nonetheless for some women it can take longer to recover their normal cycles. The NHS recommends that you allow yourself three months for a normal menstrual cycle to re-establish.

♦ **The 'mini pill'.** This contraceptive has a similar effect, thinning the uterus lining and also preventing ovulation. As soon as you stop taking it, the lining of the womb starts to thicken again and cycles re-establish. Similarly, most women recover their regular cycles after dropping the pill but in some situations the this period could be longer.

♦ **Hormonal or copper IUD.** IUDs have a mechanical effect, making the implantation more difficult. The IUD that contains hormone, is a combined treatment where the progesterone will thicken the cervical mucus and make the womb lining thinner. In both cases, cyclic menses should reestablish within a month of their removal although with the hormonal IUD, as for the pill, it could take up to three months for the menstrual cycle to return to normal.

♦ **The vaginal ring and contraceptive patch.** Both of these hormonal contraceptive methods are relatively

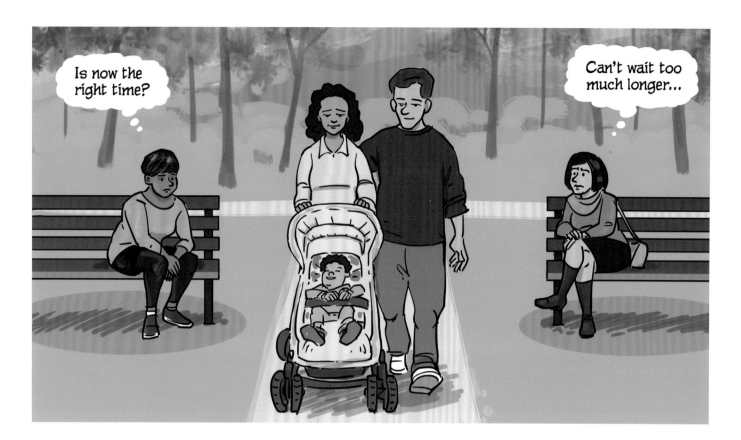

recent and so there is less research evidence on their long-term impact, but they work in a way very much like the pill, and all the evidence to date suggests that they are equally safe, and that periods return after stopping their use within the normal three months.

- **The contraceptive injection.** The 'shot' is best known in the UK under one of its trade names, Depo-Provera. The injection is repeated every three months and is especially helpful for women who don't want to be bothered with remembering to take a pill every day. However, this is the one that gives rise to all of the fears about birth control causing infertility. With this drug, it can take up to a year for your cycles to re-establish, and so it is less used among women that would like to become pregnant in the near future.

What if you don't get pregnant after stopping birth control?

A study of 2,000 women who wanted to become pregnant after taking the birth control pill for seven years was carried out by the European Active Surveillance Study on Oral Contraceptives. Researchers found:

- 21% were pregnant within one cycle after stopping birth control,

- 79% were pregnant within one year,

- Rates of pregnancy were lower among women over the age of 35.

These results reflect the chances of pregnancy in the general population, and researchers concluded that birth control has no effect on fertility. So why does the belief persist that birth control pills can cause infertility?

The explanation may be in another common misconception about birth control pills; that they make your menstrual cycle regular. They appear to, but only because the controlled levels of hormone create a 'false' regularity and bleeding. If your periods were erratic before taking the pill then once you stop, your normal, i.e. irregular, pattern will return. So it is always possible that the birth control pill was in a sense disguising an underlying problem, which could only come to light when you stop taking it.

When should I seek advice if I fail to conceive?

Don't panic if you're not pregnant in the first few months after coming off birth control. To begin with, 12 months is the normal time frame given to couples when trying to conceive. Secondly, it's possible that you're one of the people whose normal rhythm takes a while to re-establish itself. Therefore, give your body time to recover and if after that you are still not pregnant after a year, or six months if you are over 35, it's time to seek fertility advice. Likewise, don't forget that for heterosexual couples, male infertility is just as likely to be the cause as any problem with the female partner. Hence why it is important to receive a reproductive assessment is order to find out potential causes of infertility.

7 January 2020

5 ways STIs can affect your fertility

A quarter of all infertility cases are thought to be caused by an undiagnosed sexually transmitted infection.

By Dr Geetha Venkat

If you have you been trying to get pregnant for a year or more with no luck, it's normal to feel frustrated and start to worry that you might have an underlying health condition. But while eating a healthy diet, ensuring you get plenty of exercise and generally looking after your health will all stand you in better stead for improved fertility, you might not have considered your sexual health.

Nearly half a million people in the UK are diagnosed with a sexually transmitted infection (STI) every year. While STIs are upsetting and embarrassing, what many people don't realise is that some STIs can affect your fertility too. In fact, as many as a quarter of all infertility cases are thought to be linked to an undiagnosed STI.

The director at Harley Street Fertility Clinic Dr Geetha Venkat looks at the most common issues associated with STIs and fertility:

Pelvic inflammatory disease and fertility

Pelvic inflammatory disease (PID) is an infection in the upper genital tract and can be either asymptomatic or symptomatic. It is a serious condition because it can permanently damage the uterus and the fallopian tubes.

However, if PID is mild and treated early, your chances of conceiving are high. Sadly, if you have severe PID or it goes untreated, the chances of your tubes becoming blocked are higher. It's estimated that one in five women with PID have fertility problems.

Chlamydia or gonorrhoea and fertility

Both infections present absolutely no obvious symptoms at all, so you might not even realise that you're infected. Therefore, it's extremely important to get tested regularly — the longer you're infected with chlamydia or gonorrhoea, the greater the likelihood that these infections will damage your fallopian tubes and future fertility. It also means that

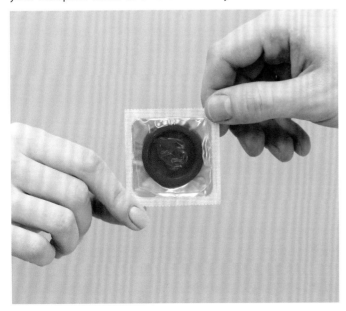

you may be inadvertently infecting a partner, impacting their future fertility as well.

Chlamydia and male infertility

It might not be the mum-to-be who has an STI. The negative impact of chlamydia on male infertility is often underestimated. Chlamydia in men can damage sperm and cause scarring in the reproductive tract (which can lead to permanent infertility). It is estimated that around 25-50 per cent of all male chlamydia cases go completely unnoticed, so get yourself checked out.

Herpes simplex virus and fertility

In most cases, the herpes virus does not affect either a woman or a man's ability to conceive. However, the biggest detriment that herpes will have on a couple's fertility is the need to abstain from intercourse during an outbreak in either partner. This can limit their chances of conceiving depending on how long the outbreak is and how often they experience flare-ups.

Fallopian tube damage and fertility

Scarring or damage to the fallopian tubes can cause what is referred to as tubal infertility. Many cases of tubal disease are caused by infection such as PID. Scarred and damaged fallopian tubes can prevent sperm from reaching and fertilising the egg.

If an egg does get fertilised, blocked tubes can also keep that fertilised egg from reaching the uterus. This can increase your odds of having an ectopic pregnancy — when the embryo implants in the fallopian tube wall, rather than in the uterus wall.

Further help and support

If you are concerned about your sexual health, it's important that you get tested. For information on where to get tested for STIs, try one of the following:

- Ask your GP for advice.
- Find a sexual health clinic near you.
- Try Brook's Find a Service tool
- Find contraceptive services near you.
- Call the national sexual health line 0300 123 7123.
- Call Worth Talking About on 0300 123 2930 (for under-18s).
- Some pharmacies also test for chlamydia.

3 September 2019

A guide to infertility

What is infertility?

Infertility (often called subfertility) is a disease of the reproductive system defined by the failure to achieve a pregnancy after 12 months or more of regular unprotected sex (without contraception) between a man and a woman. Around 9 to 15% of couples will have fertility problems. Infertility can affect men and women.

Infertility in women can be due to diverse problems. It could be a problem within the ovaries. For example eggs may be of low fertility, or ovulation may not occur, or it may occur but irregularly which would affect how often she has her period. Infertility could also be due to problems with the fallopian tubes caused by a blockage (often after infection) or with the uterus (or womb). Women can have fertility problems even if they still have regular periods.

Infertility in men is most often due to too few sperm, poor sperm quality or sperm that do not move properly.

Men's infertility could also be due to mumps when it occurs during puberty. Mumps is a viral infection that causes a swelling of glands below the ears. Finally, men can have problems ejaculating, which makes it difficult to have sex and to father a child through sexual intercourse.

Sometimes both partners can have fertility problems or sometimes the cause may be unknown. In general, approximately 30% of fertility problems are due to the woman, 30% due to the man, and 30 to 40% to both or to unknown causes.

What are the signs and symptoms of infertility?

The most obvious sign of infertility is when the woman does not get pregnant, despite having regular unprotected sex for 12 months or more (or after six cycles of insemination for same-sex couples).

Once a woman has a regular (monthly) menstrual cycle, any change in her menstrual cycle could indicate a problem. If her menstrual cycle becomes less regular, infrequent or absent then there could be a problem with ovulation. Heavier or more painful periods could be a sign of fibroids in the womb or a condition called endometriosis. Pelvic pain could be a sign of infection or endometriosis.

There are few signs for male infertility. A man usually has to have medical tests to find out if he has a fertility problem. A man's ability to have sex and ejaculate can be normal even if he has fertility problems. Men who have had mumps during puberty and men who have an undescended testis (testicle) could be at risk of fertility problems. An undescended testis means that the testis is not located in the scrotum.

If you have noticed any of the signs or symptoms mentioned in Graphic 5 or are concerned about your fertility, then talk to your doctor. The NHS 'Fertility Self Assessment tool' could also help you to decide if and when to seek help from your doctor. Fertility declines with age. Women aged 35 or older should seek help after 6 months of trying to get pregnant because if they need treatment then it is best not to delay.

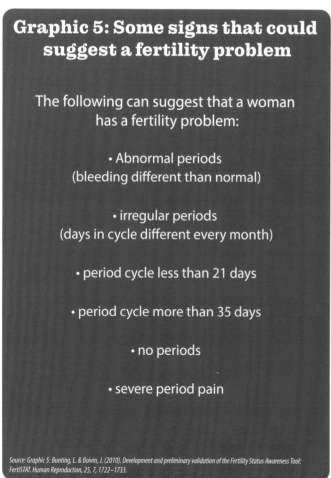

Graphic 5: Some signs that could suggest a fertility problem

The following can suggest that a woman has a fertility problem:

- Abnormal periods
(bleeding different than normal)

- irregular periods
(days in cycle different every month)

- period cycle less than 21 days

- period cycle more than 35 days

- no periods

- severe period pain

Source: Graphic 5: Bunting, L. & Boivin, J. (2010). Development and preliminary validation of the Fertility Status Awareness Tool: FertiSTAT. Human Reproduction, 25, 7, 1722–1733.

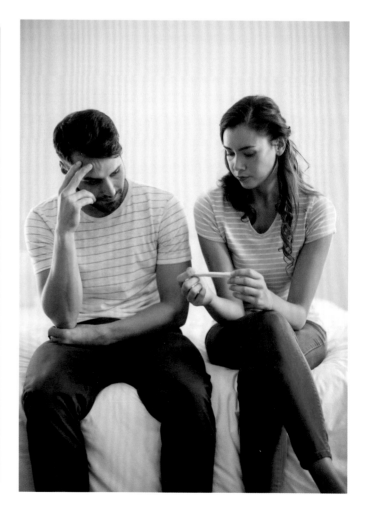

Graphic 7: Reproductive technology options

Technique	Definition	Purpose	Success rate
Contraception	• Barrier (condom) and non-barrier (hormones, coil) methods of preventing pregnancy	• Prevent pregnancy	• Highly effective, when used correctly
Medically Assisted Reproduction (MAR)	• Reproduction brought about through some form of medical intervention	• To bypass problems with fertility for example, irregular ovulation, blocked fallopian tube(s), adhesions, endometriosis, poor sperm quality • Examples include medication to stimulate production of eggs, insemination and in vitro fertilisation	• MAR can increase chance of pregnancy but can't fully compensate for age-related infertility
Use of donor eggs, sperm, embryo	• Using the eggs, sperm or embryo donated by another person or couple to have a child	• Help people with fertility problems unable to produce egg, sperm or embryos, or achieve fertilisation • Help same-sex couples or others unable to have heterosexual sex • Single women or men • People with certain disabilities • Lesbian, Gay, Bisexual, Transgender people	• Varies and depends on individual circumstance (e.g., age, type of problem) • MAR can not fully compensate for age-related infertility
Egg and sperm freezing	• Producing sperm or taking fertility drugs at a younger age to produce eggs that will be frozen now for use later at an older age.	• Postpone having children • Increase chances of pregnancy at an older age	• Varies based on age of women when freezing eggs. If freezing under age 35 better chance of future pregnancy
Surrogacy	• When a woman (the surrogate) carries and gives birth to a baby for another person or couple (the intended parents)	• For women with malformations in the womb (or after hysterectomy) or when pregnancy may be dangerous • For gay single men or couples wanting to become parents	• Good chance of success but could depend on type of surrogacy

Source: Professor Jacky Boivin, Cardiff University.

What are the main preventable causes of infertility?

There are activities that can reduce fertility. The top four activities that can affect your fertility are:

1. Being overweight with a body mass index over 25 (You can find out your body mass index on the NHS Choices website: Healthy weight calculator.)

2. Smoking especially when more than 10 cigarettes a day.

3. Having sexually transmitted infections.

4. Drinking too much alcohol – more than 6 units/week for women or 12 units/week for men. A unit is a small glass of wine, half a pint of beer or shot of spirits. Changing to a healthier lifestyle (e.g., stopping smoking and heavy drinking, or losing weight) can improve your chances of getting pregnant and of having a healthier pregnancy and baby.

What reproductive technologies are available to influence fertility?

A reproductive technology is a technique used to influence human reproduction. There are many technologies each with a different purpose.

Some of the most common techniques along with a brief description, common reasons for use, and success rates are shown in Graphic 7.

2017

www.fertilityed.uk

www.cardiff.ac.uk

9 Lifestyle factors that affect fertility

Is your lifestyle affecting your fertility?

We are all aware that factors of our lifestyle affect numerous parts of our daily lives, but when was the last time you thought 'how can my lifestyle affect my fertility?'

Never – Like many, starting a family isn't an immediate priority – but do you want children in the future? Fertility is a long-term concern. Knowing how your lifestyle can impact your fertility today, can help you when it comes to preparing to conceive in the future. It might only be a simple tweak or a change. Having a healthy lifestyle will benefit both you and your baby.

Occasionally – You are probably planning to start a family in the distant future.

Daily – You are probably planning or actively trying to start a family.

Although it isn't everything, many lifestyle factors including smoking, alcohol, BMI, certain drugs, caffeine consumption, nutrition and stress can impact your current and future fertility. This said, it should however be remembered that every individual is unique and different…and so is their fertility.

Fertility treatment is therefore not a one-size-fits-all approach. There are choices that any individual can make, to aid a healthy lifestyle and indirectly promote male and female fertility. It also takes two to tango (oocytes and spermatozoon that is), so when considering how lifestyle factors can impact on your chances of conception, all parties need to be taken into consideration.

Lifestyle factors that impact fertility:

Smoking

Smoking, be it first or second-hand smoke, can negatively impact each step of the reproductive process for both men and women. Cadmium and cotinine are two specific toxins found in tobacco smoke which can reduce sperm quality and egg production (including AMH levels). Other impacts of smoking on fertility include increased sperm DNA damage, reduced fertilisation and development potential, culminating in lower pregnancy rates.

Smoking other substances can also negatively impact fertility.

For information and help to quit smoking, please check out the services available in your local area.

Alcohol

If you're trying to conceive, the advice is not to drink alcohol at all.

If you want to reduce or stop your alcohol consumption, please contact your GP.

BMI

For both men and women, a higher or a very low BMI can impact fertility. To qualify as a private fertility patient, your BMI should be no more than 35 for men and 30 for women to be accepted as an NHS funded fertility patient.

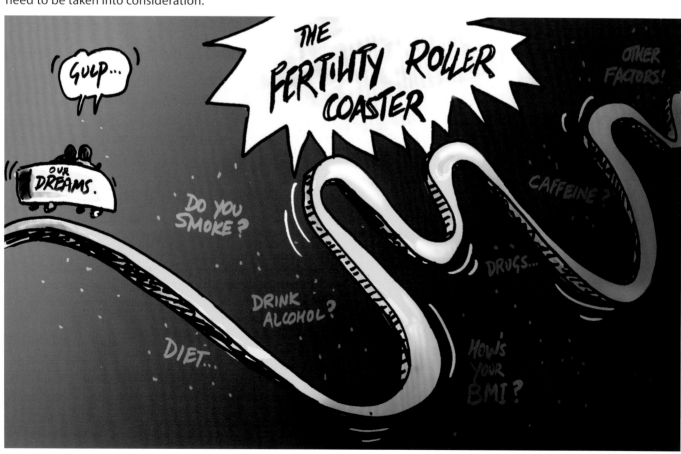

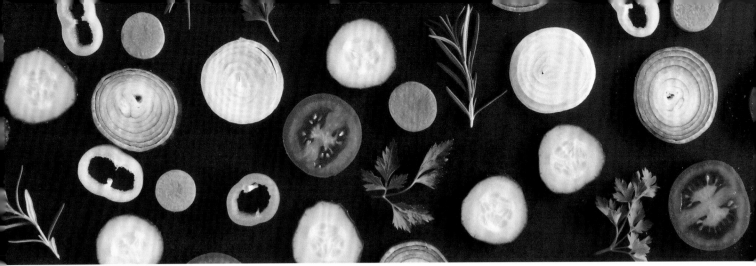

A higher BMI can impact hormonal imbalances, pregnancy risks and the amount of drugs needed for fertility treatments, in females and sperm numbers in males.

Diet

As lifestyle and fertility are connected, eating a wide variety of healthy foods is advised when trying to conceive. Eating foods, including fruits and vegetables, with antioxidant properties, are likely to be beneficial for protecting against oxidative stress, something which can be harmful to both eggs and sperm. Be mindful when consuming junk food, it should ideally be avoided. Switching from trans fats (e.g. margarine and hydrogenated vegetable oils) for unsaturated fats (e.g. oily fish and nuts) is also advised.

Exercise

Although irrelevant for most people, regular and intense exercise regimes can impact male and female fertility. Regular, moderate exercise is however proven to aid various body functions, including reproduction.

When exercising, do be mindful of taking any supplementary drugs, substances, tight underwear and your exposure to excessive heat sources (e.g. hot baths or saunas). Do seek advice from The Fertility Partnership if you are concerned that your exercise regime or occupation could be impacting your fertility.

Vitamin supplements

Wondering where to start when it comes to vitamins? We've broken down the key vitamins and supplements of interest for your fertility and all can be bought over the counter at your local chemist, in supermarkets and health stores.

Women

For female fertility, the beneficial supplements and vitamins list evolves throughout the fertility journey. Pre-pregnancy, folic acid and 'well-woman' vitamin supplements including antioxidants, Omega 3, zinc and selenium are advised. Adding in a Vitamin D (10µg/day) supplement after conception is beneficial to both a developing baby and its mother.

Taking 400 micrograms (400 µg) of folic acid to supplement your diet, pre-pregnancy and during the first 12 weeks of pregnancy, has been found to reduce the risk of developmental abnormalities.

Men

Individual vitamins and 'well-man' vitamin supplements can also be helpful for male fertility, particularly in the case of lower sperm function. Key ones to look out for include antioxidants, Omega 3, zinc and selenium.

Medication

Whether it's a one-off prescription or over-the-counter medication which you take regularly, please do consult the pharmacist, information leaflets and labels to establish the impact of your medication on your fertility. When you're trying to have a baby, there are some everyday medications that are not advised.

Contraception

It is a myth! Contraception itself, be it the pill, IUS, IUD, Injection, ring or implant, cannot make you infertile. Doctors, pharmacists and nurses actively avoid causing harm, therefore they would not prescribe contraception that had the ability to make you infertile.

Mental health

There are no ifs or buts about it…fertility is an emotional rollercoaster. It is essential that you take time to acknowledge that the stress, strains and anxiety that come with trying to conceive can't always be avoided (even with the best intentions). We strongly advise prioritising your overall health and well-being (physical and mental) when looking to conceive and whilst undergoing fertility treatment.

Patients often find establishing a strong, support network is useful for discussing their thoughts and feelings. Integrating counselling into your fertility journey can also help individuals and couples, by allowing them the opportunity to confidentially explore any feelings and distress they are experiencing.

It's all relative…

Yes, lifestyle factors can impact both an individual's and a couple's chances of conceiving…but it is all relative and, in some cases, it may be less or more than you think.

Remember you and your fertility are unique, look for fact, not fiction, and there is support out there.

6 November 2020

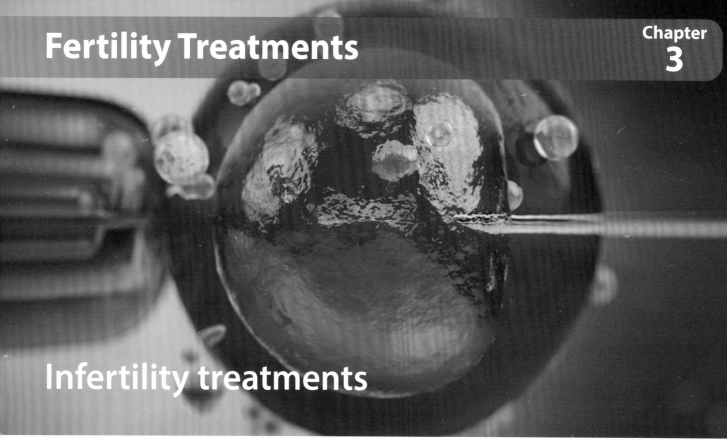

Fertility Treatments

Infertility treatments

I f you have fertility problems, the treatment you're offered will depend on what's causing the problem and what's available from your local clinical commissioning group (CCG).

There are 3 main types of fertility treatment:

♦ medicines

♦ surgical procedures

♦ assisted conception – including intrauterine insemination (IUI) and in vitro fertilisation (IVF)

Medicines

Common fertility medicines include:

♦ clomifene – encourages the monthly release of an egg (ovulation) in women who do not ovulate regularly or cannot ovulate at all

♦ tamoxifen – an alternative to clomifene that may be offered if you have ovulation problems

♦ metformin – is particularly beneficial for women who have polycystic ovary syndrome (PCOS)

♦ gonadotrophins – can help stimulate ovulation in women, and may also improve fertility in men

♦ gonadotrophin-releasing hormone and dopamine agonists – other types of medicine prescribed to encourage ovulation in women

Some of these medicines may cause side effects, such as nausea, vomiting, headaches and hot flushes.

Speak to your doctor for more information about the possible side effects of specific medicines.

Medicine that stimulates the ovaries is not recommended for women with unexplained infertility because it has not been found to increase their chances of getting pregnant.

Surgical procedures

There are several types of surgical procedures that may be used to investigate fertility problems and help with fertility.

Fallopian tube surgery

If your fallopian tubes have become blocked or scarred, you may need surgery to repair them.

Surgery can be used to break up the scar tissue in your fallopian tubes, making it easier for eggs to pass through them.

The success of surgery will depend on the extent of the damage to your fallopian tubes.

Possible complications from tubal surgery include an ectopic pregnancy, which is when the fertilised egg implants outside the womb.

Endometriosis, fibroids and PCOS

Endometriosis is when parts of the womb lining start growing outside the womb.

Laparoscopic surgery is often used to treat endometriosis by destroying or removing fluid-filled sacs called cysts.

It may also be used to remove submucosal fibroids, which are small growths in the womb.

If you have polycystic ovary syndrome (PCOS), a minor surgical procedure called laparoscopic ovarian drilling can be used if ovulation medicine has not worked.

This involves using either heat or a laser to destroy part of the ovary.

Correcting an epididymal blockage and surgery to retrieve sperm

The epididymis is a coil-like structure in the testicles that helps store and transport sperm.

Sometimes the epididymis becomes blocked, preventing sperm from being ejaculated normally. If this is causing infertility, surgery can be used to correct the blockage.

Surgical extraction of sperm may be an option if you:

♦ have an obstruction that prevents the release of sperm

♦ were born without the tube that drains the sperm from the testicle (vas deferens)

♦ have had a vasectomy or a failed vasectomy reversal

Both operations take a few hours and are done under local anaesthetic as outpatient procedures.

You'll be advised on the same day about the quality of the tissue or sperm collected.

Any sperm will be frozen and placed in storage for use at a later stage.

Assisted conception

Intrauterine insemination (IUI)

Intrauterine insemination (IUI), also known as artificial insemination, involves inserting sperm into the womb via a thin plastic tube passed through the cervix.

Sperm is first collected and washed in a fluid. The best quality specimens (the fastest moving) are selected.

In vitro fertilisation (IVF)

In vitro fertilisation (IVF), is when an egg is fertilised outside the body. Fertility medicine is taken to encourage the ovaries to produce more eggs than usual.

Eggs are removed from the ovaries and fertilised with sperm in a laboratory. A fertilised egg (embryo) is then returned to the womb to grow and develop.

Egg and sperm donation

If you or your partner has an infertility problem, you may be able to receive eggs or sperm from a donor to help you conceive. Treatment with donor eggs is usually done using IVF.

Anyone who registered to donate eggs or sperm after 1 April 2005 can no longer remain anonymous and must provide information about their identity.

This is because a child born as a result of donated eggs or sperm is legally entitled to find out the identity of the donor when they become an adult (at age 18).

Eligibility for fertility treatment on the NHS

Fertility treatment funded by the NHS varies across the UK. Waiting lists for treatment can be very long in some areas.

The eligibility criteria can also vary. A GP will be able to advise about your eligibility for treatment, or you can contact your local clinical commissioning group (CCG).

If the GP refers you to a specialist for further tests, the NHS will pay for this. All patients have the right to be referred to an NHS clinic for the initial investigation.

Going private

If you have an infertility problem you may want to consider private treatment. This can be expensive, and there's no guarantee of success.

It's important to choose a private clinic carefully.

You should find out:

♦ which clinics are available

♦ which treatments are offered

♦ the success rates of treatments

♦ the length of the waiting list

♦ the costs

Ask for a personalised, fully costed treatment plan that explains exactly what's included, such as fees, scans and any necessary medicine.

Choosing a clinic

If you decide to go private, you can ask a GP for advice. Make sure you choose a clinic licensed by the HFEA.

The HFEA is a government organisation that regulates and inspects all UK clinics that provide fertility treatment, including the storage of eggs, sperm or embryos.

Complementary therapy

There's no evidence to suggest complementary therapies for fertility problems are effective.

The National Institute for Health and Care Excellence (NICE) states further research is needed before such interventions can be recommended.

18 February 2020

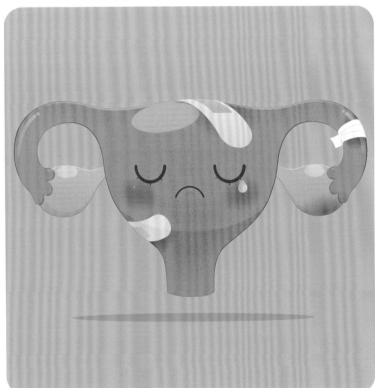

UK's IVF success rate has tripled in last 20 years

Regulator says almost a third of transfers in under-35s result in a baby but NHS funding has fallen in England.

By Helen Pidd

IVF success rates have tripled over the last 20 years in the UK, with almost a third of all embryo transfers in women under 35 resulting in a baby, according to the fertility regulator.

But patients in parts of England are finding it increasingly difficult to access NHS funding for infertility treatment due to what one expert described as a 'hugely disappointing' fall in NHS-funded cycles. Though UK guidelines say women under 40 should be given three full IVF cycles, that only happens by default in Scotland, where 60% of treatments were NHS funded in 2018, statistics from the Human Fertilisation and Embryology Authority (HFEA) show.

In England, where funding is decided by local clinical commissioning groups (CCGs), there is a postcode lottery, with just some offering three cycles and others none. Many CCGs have reduced funding for fertility treatment, with the biggest decreases seen in the east of England as well as Yorkshire and the Humber, cutting the England-wide share of NHS funded cycles to 35% from 41% in 2013.

The chances of IVF succeeding has improved across all age groups since 1998, though younger women continue to have a far higher birth rate. In 2018, the average birth rate per embryo transferred for all IVF patients was 23% – but was 31% for under-35s, compared with less than 5% for patients 43 and above when using their own eggs.

Women over 40 who use donor eggs rather than their own have a much higher chance of a baby – 25% per embryo transfer, compared with 10% when using their own eggs.

Since 2013, the number of egg and embryo storage cycles increased fivefold to just under 9,000 cycles in 2018, as freezing techniques improved and have become more commonplace.

Frozen embryo transfers are now more successful than fresh transfers, with 24.8% resulting in a baby (the birth rate from fresh transfers is 22.7%). Doctors increasingly freeze all embryos from each IVF cycle, not just the 'spares', giving a woman's body more time to get back to normal after the physically arduous process of ovarian stimulation.

Black and minority ethnic women in the UK are more likely to turn to IVF the figures show. Just 59% of all IVF cycles in 2018 were undertaken by white people, who make up an estimated 86% of the UK population as a whole.

Prof Adam Balen, the Royal College of Obstetricians and Gynaecologists spokesperson on reproductive medicine, welcomed the increased birth rates but criticised the reduction in funding, saying IVF should not be an 'easy target' for cost cutting.

'What is hugely disappointing is the continued fall in NHS-funded cycles. In 2018 in Scotland, 60% of treatment was NHS-funded, compared to 45% in Northern Ireland, 41% in Wales and 35% in England,' he said.

'Whilst the NICE [National Institute for Health and Care Excellence] guidance states that all eligible couples should be entitled to three full cycles (including the use of frozen embryos) and we know, using latest statistics, that this will give them an 80-85% chance of having a baby – and indeed many will not require the full three cycles, with on average 30% conceiving with one cycle (and in the best cases maybe 40-45%) – IVF is seen to be an easy target.

'But infertility is a serious medical condition, resulting in huge stress and distress and caused itself by a large number of different medical problems. Indeed, it is the second commonest reason for women of reproductive years to visit their GP. IVF is cost effective and has shown to be an economic benefit to society.'

Though IVF has traditionally been associated with twins, the multiple birth rate from the procedure has decreased to 8%, its lowest level since 1991, when the rate was 29.1%. This follows research proving that implanting more than one embryo does not result in a better chance of having a baby.

Implanting more than one embryo has no significant impact on the chance of a live birth but results in a 32% multiple birth rate for patients under 35.

Sally Cheshire, chair of the HFEA, said this reduction made pregnancy and childbirth much safer for women and babies.

'I am delighted that we have continued to make progress on reducing the multiple birth rate, making fertility treatment now safer than ever before. We know that multiple births are the biggest single health risk from IVF for mothers and babies and put an additional burden on the NHS.

'That's why it is a great achievement that for the first time our 10% multiple birth rate target was achieved across all age groups and nationally only 8% of IVF births resulted in a multiple birth. This shows that there is now a common understanding that implanting more than one embryo does not increase your chances of having a baby.'

30 January 2020

Going through IVF for five years, it invaded every area of my life

By Miriam Christie

There it was again. A big fat 'no'. I wasn't pregnant – and it wasn't fair. So much invested time, money and hope, to have everything dashed by a pregnancy stick.

Glen and I had started trying for a baby pretty much as soon as we got back from our honeymoon. We both knew we wanted a family and I was well aware that me being 33 meant that the clock was ticking.

After six months of trying, however, I started to worry there was something wrong. I explained the situation to my GP through a mortifying torrent of tears and was referred to a specialist, which is where our five-year journey of assisted fertility began.

Glen had a sperm test and I had a number of checks for issues with my ovaries or fallopian tubes, but nothing showed up. Part of me was relieved there was nothing obviously 'wrong' with me. On the other hand, I sort of wished there was something to fix. My infertility felt like a mystery that no one could solve.

It took nearly two years to get the green light for NHS IVF. In the meantime, I was put on a fertility drug called Clomid that bloated my stomach so much I looked pregnant. The side-glances and knowing smiles from friends and colleagues felt like a cruel irony month after unsuccessful month.

Glen and I were excited and nervous to begin with, but then our test results were misplaced, appointments were cancelled and lost in the system, or bafflingly made for a date when the consultant was on holiday. I felt like my window of time to have a baby was closing.

At our appointments, I was given a medley of injections, pills and pessaries, and a nurse showed me how to inject my stomach. Over the following 18 months, we had two frozen embryos that didn't survive the thawing stage and two failed transfers, in which specialists attempted to place embryos in the uterus.

That sentence seems shockingly small to me on the page, with its clinical talk of 'transfers' and 'thawing'. It doesn't come close to conveying the pain that comes with it. To me, these embryos were my lost babies – our dreams of starting a family slipping away.

Awash with hormones, my belly a sea of bruises, every two-week wait ended with a soul-crushing grief that had to be tucked away in a corner of my heart so that I could keep hoping and keep going.

Over the last few years of treatment, I wasn't a good friend. I felt overwhelmed with messages, calls and Facebook posts announcing baby news. I wanted to be happy for people, but I'm ashamed to admit I felt jealous and bitter instead.

What did help was speaking to a counsellor. Well-meaning friends would try to 'fix' the problem with solutions or try to talk me into a positive mood, but what I needed was to be heard.

Therapy provided me with a weekly space to talk through all of my thoughts and feelings without the brave face.

I lost touch with who I was outside of trying for a baby sometimes, so it was helpful to make time to do simple things that I enjoyed. For me, both a sweaty run and a mindful yoga practice helped to lift my mood and make friends with my body again.

The years of IVF put an incredible strain on our relationship. It was all happening to my body and I felt responsible, while Glen felt left on the sidelines and unsure how to support me. Spending time together to listen and talk about our worries helped us to reconnect and feel close when times were tough.

As I approached another birthday, we decided to try again with a private clinic. We went with one offering an Access Fertility programme that meant paying a flat fee of £10,500 for unlimited IVF cycles in London, which helped me to separate the emotional cost from the financial burden.

The process this time around was mercifully smooth and supportive but, as a result of my increasing age, just five eggs were collected, resulting in three embryos.

After another failed attempt, our second embryo became our baby. I will never forget our joy at seeing the words 'pregnant' on the test stick. After so long trying, it was a while before I could really believe it was true. Axl was born two weeks overdue by emergency C-section on 22 March 2020.

I turn 40 this December and we have one embryo left 'in the freezer', so we have a big decision to make about whether we have it in us to try again.

A legacy of my years of IVF was fear. Other mums-to-be bought baby clothes and decorated rooms, but I didn't dare make plans in case it wasn't to be.

On the other hand, I cherished the experience. I was acutely aware of how much we wanted this, how precious it was and how precarious.

Much of my work as a counsellor now is focused on supporting women through fertility issues, and the impact of pregnancy and early motherhood.

My experience has given me a deep understanding of the emotional and biological impact that IVF can have upon women. Embarking on IVF takes courage and fortitude, and there isn't always a fairy-tale ending

4 April 2021

Trying to conceive: 'I made lifestyle changes and lost five stone for IVF'

Kate Lipp and her husband Nick, who struggled to conceive for four years, overhauled their lifestyle.

By Claudia Tanner

Trying for a baby can be an emotional roller coaster, especially if you are struggling to fall pregnant as quickly as you'd hoped.

While couples can't control all of the causes of fertility issues, there are a number of lifestyle changes which can have a significant impact on the ability to conceive, including quitting smoking, getting to a healthy body weight, exercising and following a nutritious diet.

A healthy BMI is important for both partners' fertility, and if a woman's BMI is above 30, she risks being excluded from NHS-funded IVF treatment.

There is growing evidence to suggest that a typical western diet – with high intakes of processed red meat, sugar, fat, and refined grains – can impact egg quality and sperm quality.

Kate Lipp and her husband Nick had no success trying to conceive for four years, which prompted them to take stock of their poor lifestyle habits and lose 9 stone between them in the process.

Here we ask Kate, 34, now mother to three-year-old Amber, about her approach and a fertility expert for science-based lifestyle advice.

'The changes were worth it'

Kate, from Hail Weston, Cambridgeshire, was 17 stone and never exercised. She puts her weight gain down to snacking and takeaways.

After a year of trying for a baby without success, the couple went to their GP who did tests and found nothing wrong. Kate was 26 then and women aged under 40 have to have been trying for two years before NHS-funded IVF is considered.

The mobile hairdresser says it was 'frustrating' to just be told it was a 'waiting game' and not to have been given any lifestyle advice by their GP on what they could do to improve their chances. But through her their own research, the Lipps realised the importance of BMI.

So Kate lost five stone, and Nick dropped four stone. They both ensured they planned their meals ahead, ate more veg, and cut down on carbs. 'I didn't calorie count as I've never liked that,' said Kate. 'I made sure I had more veg than anything else on my plate. I ate a bit of fruit but not loads. I cut back on bread and potatoes.

'A typical day would be porridge in the morning, soup or pasta for lunch, and for dinner chicken with lots of roasted veg and tiny bit of potato or cous cous. I'd skip dessert or have some yoghurt. I was grabbing convenience food on the go at lunch time – like a pork pie, or a scotch egg – so

> ### The link between weight and fertility
>
> Overweight and obese women have higher levels of the hormone leptin, which is produced in fatty tissue, according to IVF specialist Karin Hammarberg. This can disrupt the hormone balance and lead to reduced fertility (being underweight can also throw off your hormones).
>
> Weight can also impact men's fertility: It's estimated carrying an extra 10 kilos reduces it by 10 per cent. Obesity reduces sperm quality and changes the physical and molecular structure of sperm cells.

I made sure I had a packed lunch and I always had fruit or baby cucumbers on me for snacks.'

Kate started going to the gym five times a week. 'I did a lot of weights and used the cross trainer, rowing machine and running machine – though I've got bad knee and don't run but power walk instead.'

While making a lifestyle change is important, many experts advise women to try to not get too stressed about it. 'I allowed myself a piece of cake when I fancied it, or had a few cocktails when I was on holiday,' said Kate. 'We had the attitude of whatever will be will be, though of course it was very hard when I heard about people getting pregnant.'

The Lipps were referred for NHS-funded fertility treatment at Bourn Hall in Cambridge, where they were again told they had 'unexplained infertility'. But thankfully, they fell pregnant after one cycle. 'I was actually at the gym the day I gave birth.'

Kate went to pregnancy yoga and she believes her improved fitness may have helped her have a smooth birth. And she has carried on her fitness lifestyle and since lost another two stone – taking her to just under 10 stone.

'I feel so much healthier and fitter and the changes were worth it. Amber is just brilliant, she's a madam but she keeps us smiling and laughing.'

Lifestyle recommendations

Angela Attwood, a nutritional therapist who works with Bourn Hall patients, said there is a lot that people can do to boost their fertility. 'Obviously it depends on the underlying cause of struggles with conceiving, but there's tons of factors, such as weight, diet, smoking, lack of sleep, and stress,' she said.

'There is so much that people can do before they get to needing fertility treatments that could possibly avoid the trauma involved, and lots they can do to help boost their

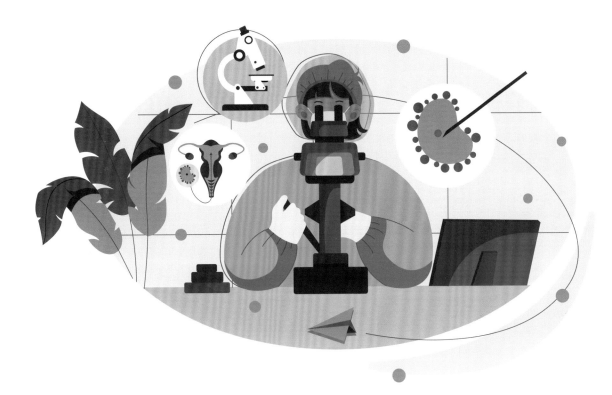

chances during treatment. And it's not just important for women but for men too.'

Stressing that advice would depend on the individual, for instance if a woman had polycystic ovary syndrome, Angela has summarised the general concepts below.

Alcohol – Alcohol affects sperm and egg health by raising free radicals in the body and depleting essential nutrients necessary for reproductive health. It's advisable to eliminate alcohol when preparing for and during fertility treatment. One study found that consumption of as few as four alcoholic drinks per week is associated with a decrease in IVF live birth rate.

Smoking – Chemicals found in cigarette smoke can increase the rate of women's egg loss and reproductive function. And we often think about the harmful impact on women, but it's a really big deal for men as well. Studies show men who smoke have lower sperm counts, decreased motility (sperm's ability to swim), fewer normally shaped sperm, and increased sperm DNA damage.

BMI – A healthy BMI is associated with improved fertility treatment success. Women with a high BMI may find it difficult to become pregnant as fat cells produce oestrogen, which may upset their hormone balance.

Carbohydrates – We know now that eating too many refined carbs is linked to increased risk of many diseases, including heart disease and type 2 diabetes. There is a growing body of evidence linking such foods to impaired fertility: A high carbohydrate intake results in raised insulin levels, which are detrimental to egg health and high carbs are also linked to obesity, which in itself reduces fertility.

Researchers at Harvard Medical School found that women who consumed around 60 per cent of their calories from carbs (compared to a 40 per cent group) had a 91 per cent higher risk of ovulatory infertility. It's not about no carbs at all, it's about reducing them and opting for 'good' carbs – whole grains, vegetables, fruits and legumes.

Mediterranean diet – Research suggests women who follow a Mediterranean-style diet high in vegetables, vegetable oils, fish and beans are more likely to increase their chances of getting pregnant. Opt for good quality olive oil, avocados, nuts and seeds. The NHS recommends a healthy, balanced diet should include at least two portions of fish a week, including one of oily fish.

Caffeine – Drinking a lot of caffeine before and during pregnancy has been linked to infertility, miscarriage and low birth weight so the general advice is for women to limit their intake to 200mg a day – approximately two cups of coffee. For those who can't go without I would recommend one cup of coffee a day max – ideally decaffeinated. Tea does have less caffeine, but again decaf, green or herbal teas are good options.

Supplements – Folic acid can significantly reduce the risk of a foetus developing neural tube defects in early pregnancy and should be taken by all women who are trying to conceive. There are a lot of other types of fertility supplements out there: some are good, some are bad, some just don't contain sufficient dosages in them. The issue is that many are not tailored to the individual. It's important to seek expert advice on supplements so they are right for you.

8 January 2021

Considering using IVF to have a baby? Here's what you need to know

An article from *The Conversation*.

THE CONVERSATION

By Hannah Brown, Chief Science Storyteller, South Australian Health & Medical Research Institute & Louise Hull, Associate Professor and Fertility and Conception Theme Leader, The Robinson Research Institute, University of Adelaide

If it's not you, perhaps it's someone you know. You don't look infertile, you don't feel infertile, but after many months (or years) of trying to start a family, followed by several months of monitoring your cycle in a fertility clinic, it's time to discuss IVF.

This is a big decision. It will impact your time, your finances, your emotions, your relationships and your dreams of being a parent.

Despite the language of 'falling pregnant', inferring absolute simplicity, infertility is a reality for one in six Australian couples.

Infertility isn't picky, but it is ageist!

A woman's age is the single best predictor of IVF success. This is because a woman is born with all the eggs she will ever have, somewhere between one and four million. Our eggs are slowly trickling out of the ovary in a steady stream, until at menopause there are no eggs left.

Despite the fact that almost 400 eggs will begin to grow each month from puberty to menopause, only one egg will survive each month, bursting out of the ovary at ovulation ready to be fertilised.

Sperm are an equally critical component of both IVF and natural fertility.

Despite the myth that male fertility is not impacted by age, a growing body of evidence shows men's age – and lifestyle factors such as excess weight, smoking and heavy drinking – affect fertility.

Intracytoplasmic sperm injection (ICSI) has been developed so fertilisation in the lab can still be successful even if only one good quality sperm is available.

What is the process and how will I feel?

IVF artificially increases the number of mature eggs ready for fertilisation. Your treatment very much depends on what your infertility diagnosis is, but for most couples undergoing IVF, the process will look a bit like this.

Step 1: ovarian stimulation

The hormone which makes eggs grow (FSH or follicle stimulating hormone) is given by very tiny, self-given injections just under the skin, in high but tailored doses. This creates a hormone tsunami, giving many eggs a chance to ride this wave.

Using IVF, we can safely increase the number of eggs the woman produces in a cycle without risking multiple births. We take the eggs out of the body, in a process known as egg harvest or oocyte pickup, or OPU. Leaving the eggs in the body for fertilisation incurs an unacceptable risk of having twins, triplets, or more.

These hormones can have some side effects, which are usually mild, and may include tenderness at the injection site, hot flashes, blurred vision, nausea, headache, irritability and restlessness. Your doctor will outline them, and tell you what to monitor.

Step 2: egg harvest (oocyte pickup)

When the eggs are mature (generally up to 18mm in size) and your estrogen levels are consistent with the egg numbers and size we need, we plan an egg harvest.

A trigger injection is given to finalise egg growth and development, and approximately 36 hours later, we perform the surgical procedure to collect them, ready to put them together with the sperm for in vitro fertilisation (IVF).

This procedure is more like a blood test than open surgery and in many units this procedure is done with pain relief while the female partner is awake. Other units use a light sedative anaesthetic, while they insert a narrow needle and camera (ultrasound) through the vagina to collect the eggs for IVF.

Step 3: in vitro fertilisation (IVF)

Over the next few hours, the embryologists will wash all the viable eggs and prepare them for fertilisation. They are then placed in a dish with thousands of sperm, which were

Live birth rate for the first IVF cycle

Proportion of live births out of total number of women undertaking their first IVF cycle by age group

<30 years	30-34 years	35-39 years	40-44 years	>44 years
43.7%	43.4%	30.5%	10.7%	1.4%

Source: Medical Journal of Australia

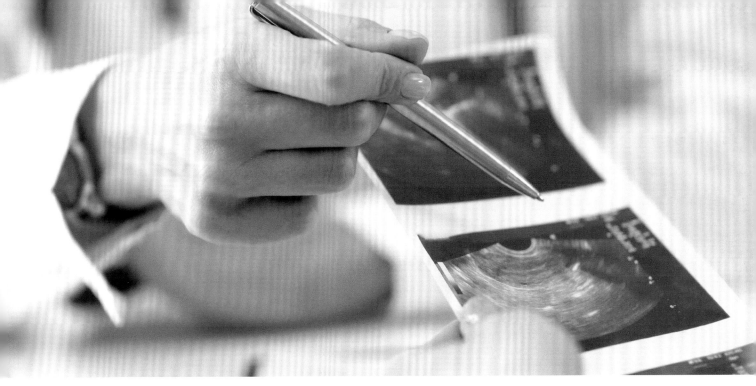

collected previously and frozen, or collected on the same day from your partner.

Step 4: embryo culture

The day after IVF, the embryologist or nurse will phone you to tell you how many eggs were fertilised.

For the next few days, your embryos will live in a dish, in an oven heated to body temperature. Staff will monitor their growth and development and will eventually pick the right one for transfer back into the womb.

The embryo is gently transferred back into the womb on day five or six, in a process similar to that of a pap test. If you have many healthy embryos at this stage, they can be frozen for use later.

Now you wait

About a week-and-a-half to two weeks after your embryo was transferred, we can test to see if it's attached to the womb. A simple blood test, or even home pregnancy test, will detect levels of human chorionic gonadotrophin (HCG), a sign that you are finally pregnant.

For some, the test will be negative. If they have frozen embryos, they can try again without needing to take more injections and have a surgical procedure.

Others will receive a diagnosis after learning something about their eggs, sperm and embryos, which can help the IVF team adjust the cycle plan and improve the couple's outcomes in future cycles.

For some, it was the last time they were going to try IVF, or fertilisation didn't occur, or an embryo transfer could not be done. Disappointment, frustration and grief becomes part of the experience and couples may need support and counselling.

For many, a positive pregnancy test is the outcome. But there is still more waiting; after all, you are still 38 weeks away from delivery. A small number of pregnancies miscarry or are lost so support in early pregnancy and good obstetric care is vital.

How much does it cost?

The cost of IVF is hugely variable, and is dependent on your level of private health cover. The out of pocket costs, even with the highest level of cover, may reach Australian $9,000* for the first cycle. And each test and process will change the price.

Sit down with your specialist and ask 'can you talk me through all of the costs associated with this round of treatment?' and have them break it down.

How do you find the right clinic?

There is a big difference in the quality of fertility care you can receive across Australia, with some clinics having dramatically higher success rates than others.

But keep in mind some clinics may not show all the data. They may quote the pregnancy rates for 'every started IVF cycle' or for 'every embryo transfer', meaning the cycles where there is no embryo to transfer are excluded – thus making the rates look unrealistically good.

Despite the desire to shop for price, asking the clinic specifically about your chance of taking home a healthy baby in their clinic, and finding a health care provider you feel comfortable with is key.

Your personal success may not be equal across two clinics, and you may save yourself money by finding a clinician and clinic with high success rates, and with a specialist who specialises in your condition, whether it's polycystic ovary syndrome (PCOS), endometriosis, or something else.

Never be afraid to ask as many questions as you have, and to ask for clarity when you don't understand. Undertaking IVF is a big step.

Costs in the UK will differ

5 February 2019

England's first not-for-profit IVF clinic to open in 2021

British Pregnancy Advisory Service is setting up fertility network to address inequalities in provision.

By Helen Pidd, North of England editor

England's first not-for-profit IVF clinic is to open in London next year, run by a charity better known for providing abortions.

The British Pregnancy Advisory Service, which has been helping women terminate pregnancies for more than 50 years, has decided to set up its own fertility network to address the inequalities in IVF provision in England.

It plans to undercut private clinics and charge only the true cost of treatment, which it estimates will be between £3,000 and £3,500 each IVF cycle, not including drugs. There will be no expensive 'add-ons' – such as embryo glue or 'assisted hatching' – which patients often feel pressured into accepting at a very vulnerable time, despite many not being proved to work.

Women should be offered three cycles of IVF on the NHS, according to guidelines from the National Institute for Health and Care Excellence (NICE), which recommends which drugs and treatments should be available on the NHS in England and Wales.

Yet IVF provision has been cut back in many areas, with some now offering no paid-for fertility treatment and others only one or two cycles. Some refuse to treat women over 35, those who cannot prove they are in a 'stable relationship' or couples with one partner who has had a child in a previous relationship.

BPAS sees parallels between the provision of IVF in 2020 with the provision of abortion in 1968, when the charity was founded.

'In 1968, women were unable to access NHS-funded abortion care and were forced to turn to private providers, who often exploited their desperation by charging extortionate prices,' said Katherine O'Brien, associate director of communications and campaigns at BPAS. 'Some private providers were also not offering an ethical service and were more akin to snake oil salesmen than medical professionals. While not as extreme as the backstreet abortions of the 1960s, it is clear that some private IVF providers are encouraging patients to undergo clinically unproven treatments at a huge personal and financial cost.'

The BPAS clinic is set to open in central London in September 2021, for egg collection and embryo transfers. Scans and other appointments will take place at satellite clinics operating from existing BPAS centres outside the capital, starting first in Peterborough and Swindon, before being rolled out across England.

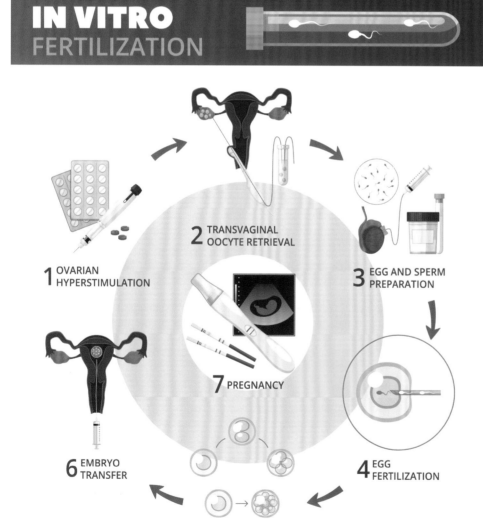

IN VITRO FERTILIZATION

1 OVARIAN HYPERSTIMULATION

2 TRANSVAGINAL OOCYTE RETRIEVAL

3 EGG AND SPERM PREPARATION

4 EGG FERTILIZATION

5 EMBRYO CULTURE FOR 2-6 DAYS

6 EMBRYO TRANSFER

7 PREGNANCY

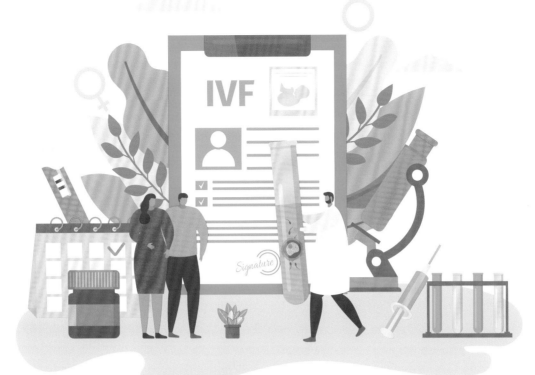

The satellite clinics will use separate entrances and different clinics for patients seeking abortions and fertility treatment, to make sure a woman wishing to terminate a pregnancy is not sitting in the waiting room next to someone desperately hoping to conceive.

It will have no set criteria for treatment, according to Marta Jansa Perez, director of embryology at the charity. 'We want our clinic to be as inclusive as possible in terms of ethnic diversity, sexual orientation and gender identities,' she said. 'We're not going to bluntly say no to anyone but we are planning to follow all professional guidelines and provide patients with the full picture in terms of chances and risks to them and the baby that they will potentially have.'

No one will be turned away for being too old, 'though we will have very honest conversations with people about their chances of conceiving and will tell them if they have next to no chance of it succeeding.'

Too many private clinics give people 'false hope', she said. People are often 'strongly pushed the hope of buying a baby' when the truth is that treatment is statistically likely to fail in many cases.

Jansa Perez had fertility treatment to conceive her two children and says she understands how vulnerable patients can be. 'I think that helps me a lot professionally, because I can see it from both sides. Even though I was successful, and I feel super privileged, I still know what it feels like,' she said.

'One of the things I feel very passionate about is that it's important that people have access to fertility treatment. It's something that impacts on people's lives quite significantly, and it impacts on people's mental health, as well.'

Like many people who have experienced infertility, she remembers 'hating seeing pregnant ladies and babies'

when she was trying to conceive. That's why the BPAS clinic and its website will not have any pictures of pregnant bellies or babies.

The BPAS clinic will start small, aiming to carry out 200 egg collections in its first year. But Jansa Perez hopes to scale it up and eventually also become a registered IVF provider for the NHS, which means some patients could choose to have their NHS-funded cycles there.

The clinic will be regulated by the Human Embryology and Fertility Authority and Jansa Perez insists it will be transparent not just in its pricing but also its success rates. Private clinics have been accused of using misleading graphs and statistics to inflate their rates, by not being clear that the data only includes women under 35, according to the fertility watchdog.

For Jansa Perez, helping patients decide when to stop treatment – or potentially not to start it in the first place – will be as important as starting it. 'A lot of patients feel that when they have a negative pregnancy test, they're either rushed on to having another treatment cycle and there is not discussion of maybe not having any further treatment, looking at the whole picture and seeing what their chances are, and whether that's something that they want to do, emotionally and financially,' she said. 'We're not selling them the baby, we're selling them a chance to possibly have one.'

29 December 2020

Surrogacy can make parenting dreams come true

A dad tells Lisa Salmon having children through surrogacy has brought him such joy, he wants to help other childless couples learn more about it.

By Lisa Salmon

Being able to have a family is something many people take for granted. But for others, it's a dream they can't achieve without help – and in increasing numbers of cases, that help is surrogacy.

If a couple can't have a baby because they have fertility issues, are the same sex, or a single man, surrogacy may be the only option, if other routes like IVF have failed or aren't possible.

Surrogacy made such a huge difference to the lives of Michael and Wes Johnson-Ellis, whose two young children were carried by a surrogate, that they started the website TwoDadsUK (twodadsuk.com) to help normalise same-sex families and destigmatise surrogacy. And now they've launched a new not-for-profit surrogacy organisation, My Surrogacy Journey (mysurrogacyjourney.com) to help other people, whether they're heterosexual or LGBTQ+, create families through surrogacy.

Here, Michael discusses their own surrogacy journey…

Michael and Wes are proud fathers to Talulah, aged four, and 18-month-old Duke, who were both carried by the same surrogate after the couple embarked on their own independent surrogacy journey.

'We went down the independent route, which meant we had to dive deeper into the communities, learn more, get informed about the law and the best clinics, and understand the independent surrogacy groups where you could meet and chat with surrogates,' explains Michael.

After huge amounts of research, the pair met the woman who was, in the end, to carry both their children, were matched with an egg donor – an anonymous woman – and embryos were created at a Manchester fertility clinic using Michael's sperm.

'Ours were donor eggs, so our surrogate didn't use her own eggs,' explains Michael. 'She'd actually been sterilised, but she wanted to carry and was adamant about doing a sibling journey for us. I'm the biological father to our daughter, and my husband is the biological father to our son.'

The couple's surrogate, Caroline, says: 'I felt that as a woman who easily falls pregnant and is usually fit and healthy during pregnancy, I had a gift to offer a couple who wouldn't

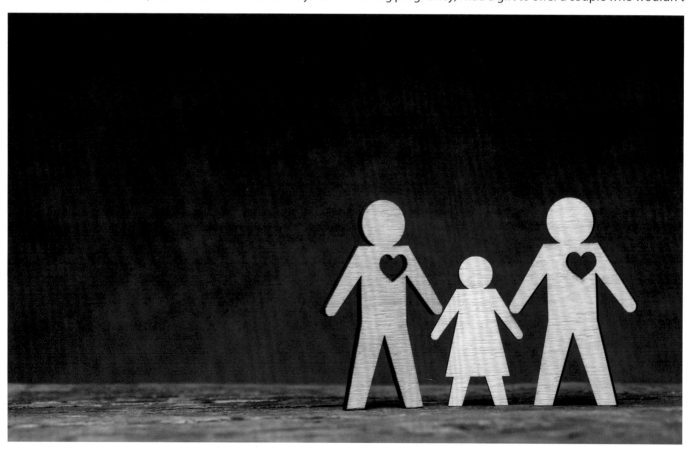

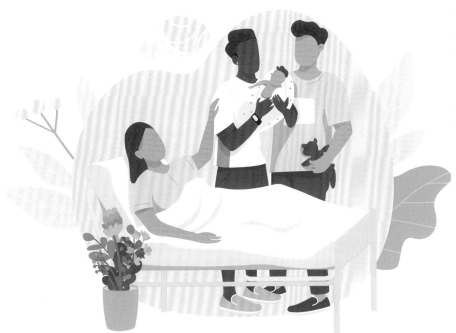

UK (surrogacyuk.org) estimates they can be anything from around £7,000 to £15,000, depending on the surrogate's circumstances and covering things like loss of earnings, childcare, maternity clothes, travel costs etc. It's also estimated that the entire cost of surrogacy for the IPs, including surrogate expenses, can be around £20,000 for straight surrogacy (where the surrogate's own eggs are used), and £30,000 for host surrogacy (where donor eggs are used and an embryo is implanted through IVF).

It's an expensive business, but it's more than worth it, says Michael. 'True surrogates don't do this to make money, this is done for the absolute gift that being a surrogate is, creating that family and seeing it. Surrogates play an incredible role in building a family, and in the majority of cases, they get a sense of achievement and pride in what they've done, to see how a family's flourishing.'

The Johnson-Ellis family see their surrogate two or three times a year, but she's not involved with the upbringing of the children. 'That's not what surrogates do,' stresses Michael, 'but she's incredibly visible and we have full disclosure to our children how they came into this world. That's what surrogates usually want.

'There will always be people who disagree with surrogacy and you have to respect their viewpoint,' says Michael cautiously, 'but I think it's really important to understand that surrogacy in the UK is built on friendship and trust. Sometimes the negativity is down to people not fully understanding that.

'Surrogacy has given us the family we'd always dreamed of, and a life we never really thought existed for two gay men. The help of donors and surrogates has enabled us to have our dream of being parents, and regardless of our sexuality, this is about people wanting to be parents, and that's everyone's right.

'Surrogacy has completely transformed not only our lives, but also our families – it's given our family members a reason to continue. The joy our children bring their extended family is the beauty of surrogacy – it creates these huge ripples and touches so many people, just by us being allowed to be parents.'

26 February 2021

otherwise have the chance to be parents. I set out wanting to create a child for a childless couple, but it's turned out to be so much more than that. I've created a family, and in doing so, changed the life of two people, but also contributed to changing the path of surrogacy in this country.'

Michael says he and Wes always wanted to educate people about surrogacy, and after setting up TwoDadsUK in 2017, thought there was more they could do.

During their own surrogacy journey, they met fertility nurse specialist Francesca Steyn, who ended up donating the eggs that helped create the couple's son, Duke.

Steyn is also a co-founder of My Surrogacy Journey, and says: 'Surrogacy is growing at a rapid rate, and each year more and more surrogacy cases take place worldwide. It's extremely successful, as you often have no fertility problems, and good egg and sperm quality. Data from the US shows a success rate of approximately 75%.'

But what about the popular belief that some surrogates will want to keep the baby they've carried, even if it's not biologically theirs?

'In my experience, surrogates never have a problem passing the child over to the parents – the intended parents [IPs],' says Steyn. 'I don't know of any cases where the surrogate has changed her mind, and we ensure IPs and surrogates have legal advice to ensure they're aware of all the legalities.'

And Michael adds: 'We think the number of cases where the surrogate has wanted to keep a child is very small. It's also important to flip that around, as sometimes surrogates have the same fear – what if the intended parents don't want the child, what if they split up, will the surrogate potentially be left with a child they don't want? I think that's equally rare, but it's interesting to look at both sides of the coin.'

Surrogates are paid expenses – although the law clearly states it's not a commercial arrangement – and Surrogacy

Surrogacy: 'Why I carried a baby for complete strangers'

Maddie Mawditt is one of five mums featured in documentary series The Surrogates, which airs on BBC3 on Sunday

By Claudia Tanner

Ask any woman who's been pregnant and she is likely to tell you it isn't all roses. There's the morning sickness, fatigue, stretch marks, followed by the actual birth.

But mothers will say it's all worth it as you get to take home your baby at the end.

Except, for Maddie Mawditt, that wasn't the plan. As soon as baby Hannah – conceived using her own eggs – was born, she was handed to her two dads, Alex and Richard Margerison, who held her with tears streaming down their cheeks.

Becoming a surrogate was 'something I'd always considered', says Maddie, 31, from Bristol, who was a single mother, with two boys, aged 10 and eight, when she started the process.

'As I was approaching my 30th birthday, I thought it was a good time to look into it; it was a now-or-never type thing. The more I found out about it, and how it's done in the UK, the more it seemed like something I really wanted to do.'

Maddie, who gave birth in July, was driven by the power of being able to make such a difference to a couple's life.

'I think wanting to have children is kind of primal, and to not be able to do something you want so much is probably one of the worst feelings ever.

'In a kind of selfish way, to be a beacon of light and have a special place in someone else's family is an amazing thing to be part of.'

'So much love in the room'

She explains that handing over the baby wasn't hard. 'As soon as she came out it was the most amazing feeling ever, just incredible.

'They put her on a towel on my tummy and Alex and Richard were frozen. I grabbed their hands and handed Hannah over. They were crying. I just had this massive grin on my face. We were all on cloud nine.'

Richard, a teacher, says: 'Having kids is something that we always, always wanted to do. Maddie made our dream come true.'

Maddie adds: 'The midwife said, 'I've never felt so much love in a room before.' And that was really lovely to hear.'

A 'dating' type experience

Alex, 38, Richard, 37, and Maddie met through SurrogacyUK, the leading UK not-for-profit surrogacy organisation, at one of their social events.

Once intended parents and a surrogate have a mutual interest in each other, they move on to a 'getting to know each other better' stage, for a recommended minimum of three months. So the trio, and Maddie's sons and new partner Amber, spent a lot of time together, including days

> ### Jon Snow welcomes baby boy via surrogate
> This week, the Channel 4 News presenter, Jon Snow, 73, announced the arrival of a son with his wife, Dr Precious Lunga, 46, via a surrogate. In a statement, Jon said: 'In our desire to seal our now 11 years of marriage with a baby, my wife suffered numerous medical setbacks and miscarriages.
> 'Consequently, we will always be deeply grateful to our surrogate, who carried our embryo to term. Amid these challenging times, we feel doubly blessed to be able to celebrate our good fortune.'

out and takeaways. They even enjoyed a holiday together. 'It felt a bit like dating,' says Maddie.

They all felt that going through an agency appealed to them as there was more structure and it felt like they were better safeguarded than organising the surrogacy independently.

Minimising risk of disputes

Surrogacy is often described as an ethical and legal minefield. Under UK law, the surrogate who gives birth is always treated as the mother and has the legal right to refuse to hand over parental rights after the birth, even if not genetically related.

Did Alex and Richard worry about this? 'We thought that was going to be a concern at the start,' says Alex, a chartered engineer from Amersham, Buckinghamshire, who has been with Richard for 19 years.

> There's trust on both sides. We'd become such close friends worrying about differences wasn't even a consideration
>
> – Alex Margerison

'But by the time we had our agreement session, we'd been getting to know Maddie for the best part of six months and seeing each other every couple of weeks. So we knew each other really well.

'And there's trust on both sides. She has to put trust in us that we're not going to get her pregnant and say, 'Sorry, we don't want this any more.' But at that point, we'd become such close friends, it wasn't even a consideration.'

Alex, Richard and Maddie met with an advisor from SurrogacyUK to devise a surrogacy agreement. It is not legally binding on the parties involved, but it's a starting point for resolving and, ultimately, preventing disputes happening in the first place.

'It covers pretty much everything that you could possibly think of, including how much contact you expect to have with each other during all the stages of pregnancy and after the birth. Who will be in the room and who will hold the baby,' says Alex.

'It looks at how you would approach any problems with pregnancy or the baby, such as whether you would terminate if the baby had Down's Syndrome. That really helps you work through if you're compatible. And with Maddie, we were totally on the same page.'

'We are like one big happy family'

After Alex and Richard met Maddie in October 2018, it took eight months for Hannah to be conceived. 'I found that quite challenging,' says Maddie. 'I thought, my goodness, have I promised them a baby and got their hopes up and can I fulfil this?'

Lockdown has severely limited how much time the two families have spent together. But they keep in touch regularly. 'It has been really sad missing out on Hannah's early development,' says Maddie. 'But Alex and Richard have kept me in the loop with pictures and video calls.'

They way we explained it to my children is that Hannah is like their cousin

– Maddie Mawditt

Boundaries regarding each other's roles have always been clear from the start. 'When it comes to decisions about Hannah's life, that was always going to be solely down to Alex and Richard,' says Maddie.

'The way we explained it to my children, which I think is a good way to look at it, is that Hannah is like a cousin. My kids just adore Alex and Richard and easily fell into calling them Uncle Alex and Uncle Richard. We are like one big, happy family.'

Richard adds: 'We are eternally grateful to Maddie. And Amber, too, who met Maddie halfway through this process, was supportive and helped Maddie while she was heavily pregnant.'

11 March 2021

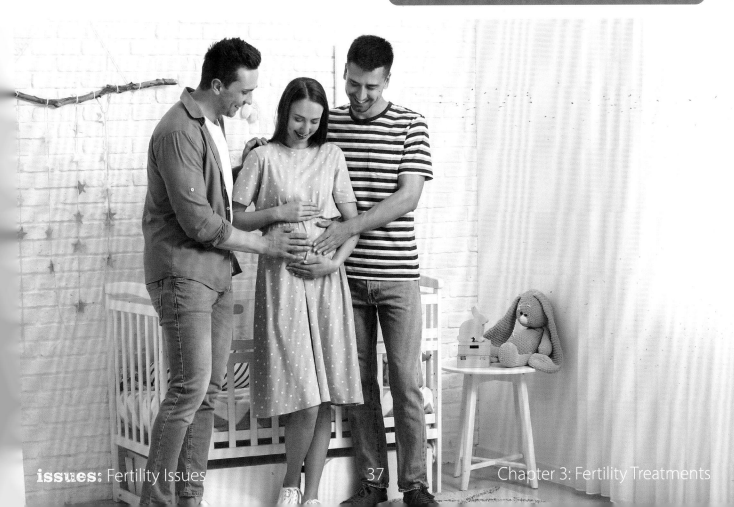

Can 'known' donors show us the future of egg and sperm donation?

By Petra Nordqvist, Leah Gilman and Hazel Burke

In common parlance, being an egg or sperm donor means donating anonymously via a clinic or bank. This group of donors are often referred to as 'ID-release donors' because, since 2005, their identity can be released to any child conceived via their donation when they turn 18.

However, alongside ID-release donation, there is also the option of 'known' donation. This is where men and women agree to act as donors for friends, family members or people they meet on social media or on donor matching platforms.

Official UK bodies such as the HFEA and the SEED Trust tend to discourage any known donation that circumvents the use of a licensed clinic. Nevertheless, it has become a widespread practice, with the internet playing an increasingly important role in donors and recipients finding each other.

As sociologists at the University of Manchester, our research on the experiences of being an egg or sperm donor has given us insights into the everyday lives of a wide variety of donors in the UK, including known donors. Our research interviews tell us something important about what it means to be a donor. Three main points stand out.

1. Donors are guided by a strong moral sense that donors should 'know their place'.

This applied to known donors who knew their offspring, as well as ID-release donors. Andy, a known donor who had donated to friends of friends, was typical in the way that he approached being a donor. He said that following the birth: 'I wanted to leave it a few weeks, so probably four or five weeks, so as to give the child plenty of time to bond with the mums…showing that I don't want to be intrusive, I want to respect that they're a family unit.' The quote shows how donors in the study saw their role as very different from the role of a parent.

The vast majority of donors we spoke to were very thoughtful about their role as donors and took particular care not to overstep the boundaries of the recipient families, allowing the parents and the donor conceived child to define and drive the relationship.

2. Donors often feel a strong link or connection to the recipient and their family.

While they do not see themselves as a parent, donors often feel a strong link or connection to the recipient and

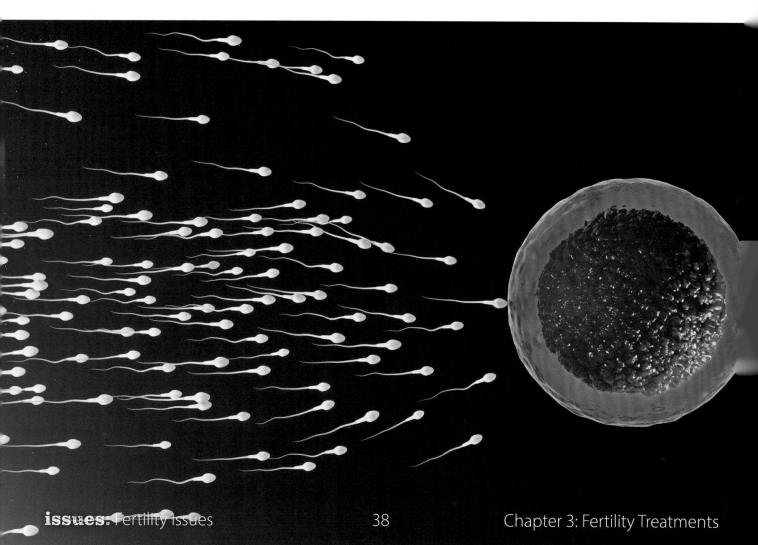

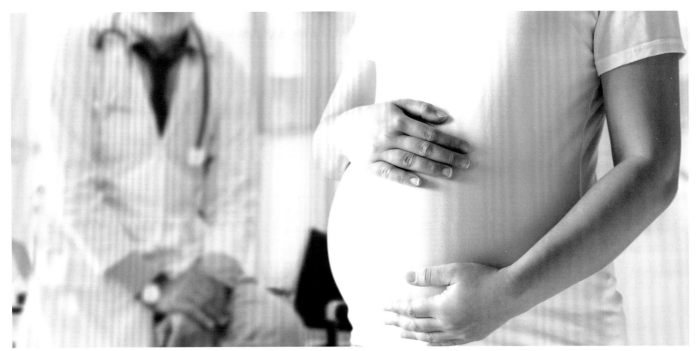

their family, without that connection being defined in any particular way. We saw a huge range in the degree of contact that known donors had with their recipient families.

As suggested in our first point, this was usually driven by the recipients. For example, in the case of Ian who had donated sperm to several families via a donor matching platform, he had no face-to-face contact with some couples after the donation, but had occasionally visited other families and kept in touch via Facebook. An egg donor, Eliza, had donated to a friend and found that the donation deepened their relationship.

So, while being a donor is not the same as being a parent, we found a real sense that the connection that comes with being a donor matters.

3. Donor relationships can shift and change over time.

As with any human relationship, known donor relationships can change quite dramatically over time. We found that when things went well, the relationships that grew between donors, recipients and their children were felt to be deeply enriching, positive and joyous. Beth, for example, who had found her recipients via an online platform, said: 'It brings me so much pleasure to know'.

By the same token, when relationships took a nosedive, they were felt to be anxiety-provoking, even toxic, and sometimes led to a devastating sense of 'heartbreak'. It is important to understand that in known donation, donors (or recipients or donor conceived people for that matter) are not solely in charge of how relationships unfold over time; as with any human relationship, it depends on the people involved, on how they get on and on how they understand their roles and responsibilities. Our data indicated that problems tended to emerge when there were discrepancies in how the various parties understood their roles and the boundaries of the relationships.

We think that taking on board these experiences could help expand the support available to all donors and recipient families in the future. This is because under the current regulatory system there is no truly anonymous donation in the UK anymore.

The 2005 law change to ID release donation (as reported in *BioNews 302*) stipulates that donor conceived young people can trace and contact their donor when they turn 18. We are now quickly approaching 2023, when the first cohort of donor conceived children will reach this legal threshold. This means that ID release donation is essentially known donation waiting to happen. However, the key difference here is that donors and recipients have never met and at no stage prior to conception have they 'chosen' (or refused) each other based on personal knowledge.

Our findings about what it is like to be a known donor show that important questions might emerge in the future when ID release donation transitions to known donation. How will donor conceived people, donors and recipients understand their connection to one another? What kind of relationship will grow between people connected through donation? What happens when people disagree on the terms of their relationship?

As 2023 is approaching, it is time to start to recognise that ID release is a form of (delayed) known donation, and that it is time to start thinking about how to make the transition a success.

9 March 2020

Key Facts

- the chance of pregnancy if people have sex -2 days before ovulation is 26% compared to 1% if they have sex +1 day after ovulation. (page 1)

- At birth, most girls have about 2 million eggs, at adolescence that number has gone down to about 400,000, at age 37 there remain about 25,000. By age 51 when women have their menopause they have about 1000 immature eggs but these are not fertile. (page 2)

- Men's fertility also starts to decline around age 40 to 45. (page 2)

- The perimenopause is a natural stage of life that occurs as you age. In most people it will happen naturally between the ages of 45 and 60, and last for a few months to several years. (page 7)

- The average age of the natural menopause is 51 years. (page 8)

- The total fertility rate (TFR) for England and Wales decreased from 1.70 children per woman in 2018 to 1.65 children per woman in 2019. (page 11)

- The standardised mean age of mother at childbirth was 30.7 years and has been gradually increasing since 1973 when it was 26.4 years. (page 12)

- For women less than 35 years of age, who have normal ovarian reserve, 30-35% percent of IVF cycles will lead to the live birth of a baby. For women aged 38 to 40, the success rate drops to almost half. Very few women aged 43 to 44, will have a live birth using their own eggs. (page 14)

- Nearly half a million people in the UK are diagnosed with a sexually transmitted infection (STI) every year. (page 19)

- Around 25-50 per cent of all male chlamydia cases go completely unnoticed. (page 19)

- Around 9 to 15% of couples will have fertility problems. (page 20)

- Approximately 30% of fertility problems are due to the woman, 30% due to the man, and 30 to 40% to both or to unknown causes. (page 20)

- Women aged 35 or older should seek help after 6 months of trying to get pregnant. (page 20)

- IVF success rates have tripled over the last 20 years in the UK, with almost a third of all embryo transfers in women under 35 resulting in a baby. (page 26)

- Black and minority ethnic women in the UK are more likely to turn to IVF. (page 26)

- Infertility is the second commonest reason for women of reproductive years to visit their GP. (page 26)

- women who consumed around 60 per cent of their calories from carbs (compared to a 40 per cent group) had a 91 per cent higher risk of ovulatory infertility. (page 29)

- Under UK law, the surrogate who gives birth is always treated as the mother and has the legal right to refuse to hand over parental rights after the birth, even if not genetically related. (page 36)

- While surrogacy is legal in the UK, no payment is allowed other than 'reasonable expenses'. You cannot pay a surrogate in the UK, except for their reasonable expenses, which can be from anywhere between £7,000 and £15,000. (page 37)

- In the US, where it is commercialised, surrogates typically receive compensation of $30,000 to $60,000. (£21,600-£43,200). (page 37)

- Since 2005 a donors identity can be released to any child conceived via their donation when they turn 18. (page 38)

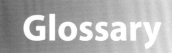

ART/Artificial Reproductive Technology

'Fertility treatments': achieving pregnancy through artificial means.

Birth rate

The number of live births within a population over a given period of time, often expressed as the number of births per 1,000 of the population.

Contraception

Anything which prevents conception, or pregnancy, from taking place. 'Barrier methods', such as condoms, work by stopping sperm from reaching an egg during intercourse and are also effective in preventing sexually transmitted infections (STIs). Hormonal methods such as the contraceptive pill change the way a woman's body works to prevent an egg from being fertilised. Emergency contraception, commonly known as the 'morning-after pill', is used after unprotected sex to prevent a fertilised egg from becoming implanted in the womb.

Donor/donor rights

A donor is someone who donates either their eggs (female) or sperm (male) to be used in fertility treatments to help people who are unable to have children of their own. Donors used to remain completely anonymous, but in 2005 the law changed so that when donor-conceived children reach 18, they can find out the identity of the donor and whether they have any half-brothers or sisters (though this largely depends on whether they are ever told they are donor-conceived).

Fertility/infertility

According to doctors, infertility is when a couple are unable to become pregnant despite having regular, unprotected sex for two years. There are a number of possible reasons for couples to be infertile. For example, a male's low sperm count, damage to a female's fallopian tubes, etc.

Fertility treatment

A medical procedure or treatment intended to increase the chance of a person conceiving a child.

Genetic testing

This refers to a technique called pre-implantation genetic diagnosis (PGD). This allows parents to test for serious genetically inherited conditions such Huntington's disease or cystic fibrosis. There is a fear that genetic testing will be misused. However, it can be legally carried out if it is in the best interest for the embryo.

IVF (In vitro fertilisation)

IVF literally means 'fertilisation in glass', giving us the familiar term 'test tube baby'. IVF treatment is considered by couples who are having fertility problems and are not getting pregnant. Eggs are removed from the ovaries and fertilised with sperm in a laboratory dish before being placed in the woman's womb (a technique where the egg is fertilised by sperm outside of the body).

Menopause

Is the permanent end of a woman's menstrual cycle; she will no longer have periods or be able to become pregnant.

Menstruation

Menstruation, or period, is the bleeding that occurs as part of a woman's monthly cycle.

Perimenopause

Perimenopause is when a woman's fertility declines, and menstruation occurs less regularly in the years leading up to the final menstrual period, when a woman stops menstruating completely and is no longer fertile.

Secondary infertility

Secondary infertility is when a couple has difficulty getting pregnant after they have conceived a child naturally in the past.

Sexually transmitted infections (STIs / STDs)

A sexually transmitted infections (STIs), also referred to as sexually transferred diseases (STDs), is a bacterial or viral infection that is spread through sexual contact. This doesn`t just mean vaginal/anal sexual intercourse, but also oral sex (licking/sucking on someone`s genitals) and sexual touching (skin-to-skin contact). Using condoms are the best way of avoiding STIs. Although STIs are treatable, if left unchecked and untreated they may cause serious damage to long-term health, such as infertility. The most common STI in the UK is chlamydia.

Surrogacy

When a couple who are unable to conceive naturally find another woman, known as the surrogate, to carry and give birth to their baby. Surrogacy is legal in the UK, but it is illegal to pay for the service. It is legal, however, to pay towards reasonable expenses such as medical costs.

Activities

Brainstorming

- In small groups, discuss what you know about fertility.
  - What age is a person most fertile?
  - What kinds of things can affect a person's fertility?
  - What is the menstrual cycle?
  - What is the difference between perimenopause and menopause?
  - What is IVF?
  - Can you think of any other fertility treatments?

- Create a Diamond9 with the things that can affect a person's fertility. Place the most important factors at the top, moving down to the least important at the bottom.

Research

- Choose a country and investigate its laws surrounding fertility treatment and surrogacy. Write a short essay, summarising your findings.

- Research the different causes of infertility, in both men and women, and make a bullet point list. Share your findings with your class.

- Research things that may affect your fertility – consider both positive and negative factors.

- Conduct a survey throughout your year group to find out how many young people have thought about their fertility and considered whether they will want children in the future. Ask at least three different questions and create a series of graphs to demonstrate your findings.

Design

- Design a leaflet that explains the risks and benefits of IVF treatment.

- Design a poster with some myths about fertility. Make sure you include the facts!

- Choose one of the articles in this book and create an infographic to display the key points of the article.

- Choose one of the articles in this book and create an illustration to convey the key theme.

- Using the article 'Our complete calendar guide to periods and the menstrual cycle', create a poster to explain the menstrual cycle.

- Design a leaflet about Perimenopause. Include symptoms and tips for women who may be experiencing perimenopause.

Oral

- With a partner, discuss the emotional and physical effects that infertility can have on couples. Consider both female and the male perspective. Make some notes and feed back to your class.

- Choose an illustration from this topic and, in pairs, discuss what you think the artist was trying to portray with this image. Does the illustration work well with its accompanying article? If not, why not? How would you change it?

- Create a PowerPoint presentation that will explain the issue of fertility to young people and highlight some things they should do to safeguard their fertility for the future.

- As a class, discuss whether you think IVF should be fully funded for people who are infertile. One half of the class should be for and the other against.

Reading/writing

- Read the article 'Can "known" donors show us the future of egg and sperm donation?'. Imagine that you had to write a letter to a donor parent – what would you include?

- Watch the 2013 film 'Delivery Man'. The main character is a donor parent to a large amount of children. Write a newspaper article imagining that this was a true story.

- Often, people who are suffering from fertility problems don't speak to friends and family about what they are experiencing. Write a letter to an agony aunt/uncle where you can say your worries about not conceiving. Then, write a reply offering advice.

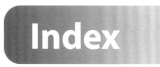

Acknowledgements

The publisher is grateful for permission to reproduce the material in this book. While every care has been taken to trace and acknowledge copyright, the publisher tenders its apology for any accidental infringement or where copyright has proved untraceable. The publisher would be pleased to come to a suitable arrangement in any such case with the rightful owner.

The material reproduced in *ISSUES* books is provided as an educational resource only. The views, opinions and information contained within reprinted material in *ISSUES* books do not necessarily represent those of Independence Educational Publishers and its employees.

Images

Cover image courtesy of iStock. All other images courtesy of Pixabay and Unsplash.

Illustrations

Simon Kneebone: pages 10, 14 & 22. Angelo Madrid: pages 5, 12 & 18.

Additional acknowledgements

With thanks to the Independence team: Shelley Baldry, Danielle Lobban, Jackie Staines and Jan Sunderland.

Tracy Biram

Cambridge, May 2021